SUGAR WILL KILL YOU

There are no pizzas, tacos, cheeseburgers, ice cream, French fries, fried chicken, doughnuts, and all the tasty foods in heaven. None of the religious books mentions these foods, and that is why Jesus wants to come back, and Adam left the garden because they were tired of eating the milk, honey, grapes, and dates. These, after all, are just full of sugars, so what exactly are we going to heaven for?

Even though I was taught that there are bad fats and good fats, I do not believe that anymore because all fats are made out of carbon, hydrogen, and oxygen. The only difference they have are the sources they come from, the chemical bonds between the carbon and the hydrogen atoms, and the way they are preserved by humans. All fats produce nine calories per gram of fat. Furthermore, through my years of being brainwashed in schools, I learned that eating fats, especially saturated fats from animal products, cause heart diseases, diabetes, and promote major health risks, but I find this information to be misleading. Fats don't make you fat.

It is the lack of discipline and ignorance from the person who eats. Ironically, I eat fatty foods such as fried chicken, fish, cheese, pizza, butter, and French fries. I find these foods to be tasty and appealing. Part of what makes them tasty is the fat while all the foods that are supposedly good for you taste horrible.

After eating fatty foods, my brain memory and signal, reception improves tremendously, and they allow my body to easily absorb certain vitamins and supplements. Eating fatty foods generates good energy, which helps my heart and lungs when I'm jogging and running for long distances. In addition, fats give me shiny skin and protect me from the excessive rays of the sun. Of course, fats also increase my libido and testosterone levels and makes me salivate for those pretty women out there, especially those with a little cushion. My body needs certain levels of fats, and there is nothing wrong with them as long as I burn the excess fats by jogging, walking, lifting weights, resting, and drinking lots of water. It is all a natural process.

There is a private party in nature called photosynthesis where the sun, water, carbon dioxide, and plants become friends and want to have a good time, so they create an addictive drug called sugar, which is made out of Carbon, hydrogen, and oxygen. Sugar thus is a necessary part of nature. These three groupies enjoy getting tipsy, and then the uninvited party poopers of humanity showed up at the party. They stole the sugar formula and turned it into the greatest drug business ever. Humans are simply robbing the plants of their natural product.

We cannot produce sugar of our own, and people do not realize that sugar is a part of everything we eat. Sugar molecules hold our own DNA together. It is a part of our genetic makeup, which is life itself. It is a part of all living things.

Food affects mood in a more powerful way than people realize. As with all things in life, we have to pace ourselves and monitor our in-take of certain foods. I spoke with many of my students who suffer from diabetes, heart diseases, liver diseases, cancer, and depression, and all of them shared with me these serious health problems come from eating foods and drinks loaded with sugars and high fructose corn syrup. In addition, these students are not active, nor do they exercise to burn the deadly triglyceride fats that cause inflammation and poison our bodies. They also shared with me that their insulin levels spike and cause them to be hungry all the time.

When insulin levels rise, it turns on the leptin hormone. This hormone is a signal that controls our hunger levels, and it controls the floodgates of feeling hungry. High insulin levels keep this switch set to "On." As a result, people in this state feel hungry all the time, and in fact, they are not physically hungry but are psychologically hungry. Their metabolism eventually slows down because they are still absorbing calories they do not need. Once the body is unable to convert all the calories, it will start gaining more weight.

The body eventually becomes insulin resistant, and there will be more glucose floating in the blood. As the weight gain mounts, there will be lots of pressure on the heart to function fully. A person in this condition will find his or herself tired all the time, and before they know, they are in a diabetic condition.

This behavior of loving sugar may eventually lead to liver, pancreas, and heart and kidney diseases. Once the major body organs functions are affected, the chances of continued survival are slim.

I eat carbohydrates such as breads, yams, pasta, and corn because I run and jog a lot, and my muscles and brain need these sugars to burn for energy. I also know that some of the carbohydrates that I eat will be converted into glycogen as a reserve for later use, and I minimize my consumption of refined foods. When you eat foods or drink drinks that have excess sugars, your insulin level will spike which eventually causes a traffic jam in your body, the building block of which is the cell. Your cells can only absorb and process so much, so when there is excess fuel, they eventually stop absorbing and metabolizing these materials.

These products then sit without use, and they eventually become toxic. These toxins drift through the blood stream to the brain, heart, liver, and kidneys. The infected blood eventually reaches every organ, but this is not the only negative effect.

The body does not only shut off its absorption of excess sugars. It also blocks the absorption of minerals, calcium, potassium, and iron. These are key substances that your body needs to operate in an efficient and healthy manner. The body soon becomes intoxicated, and it has a similar effect as a night of heavy drinking.

People often complain about headaches, fatigue, malaise, and other issues. They do not even realize it is the result of eating sugary foods. There are many misconceptions about nutrition, health, and fitness. The food industry and pharmaceutical companies intentionally put out this misinformation to keep people in the dark and confused. Naturally, this is done to the detriment of people's health in order to make more money.

AMERICAN BUSH GIRL

I stayed at the college and never went clubbing or got involved in drugs. I was there to finish my PhD. They had a ballroom in which they had dance nights on Fridays. I started to attend. I was raised where people dance and play drums. I wanted to dance and enjoy the music at the ballroom, which was not that great. There was no bush girl to dance with because every woman there was white. All the skinny white ladies were taken, and only a few chubby ones were left. I was desperate, and it was wintertime.

I needed a woman to keep me warm through the long winter nights. A man has to have a woman no matter what. I tried desperately to meet every woman on and outside the dance floor.

I encountered a few rejections, but finally, a five feet seven-inch brunette said that she would dance with me. I got down with her, and she liked the way I moved. I always had a variety of moves, and this comes from my African heritage.

"What's your name?" she asked.

"I'm Ali."

"I'm Jennifer." She had large beautiful eyes, big titties, and a nice ass, which made my mind race to all the wrong places. She had jungle fever, and I fevered her up in the bushes. She became my American bush girl: uh uh uh, hear me roar…

We danced together for a long time, and got to know each other.

She said, "Do you like country music? Would you like to go with me to a rodeo?" I had never danced to country music, but she made me an even more desperate man, so I said, "Yes."

I bought a cowboy hat, boots, and turned out to be a good looking, tall black cowboy. I went to the rodeo, and danced to a country music song for the first time, and I figured out immediately how to dance to country because there is not much to it. I took her to a Ziggy and Steven Marley concert in Park City, Utah because she took me to a country show.

She told me that she liked me, and I said I liked her too. I met her family, and they liked me as well. She would take me to the bushes of Utah where nobody would see us. She also taught me how to match my clothes because I never knew or heard about matching. We dated until I left Utah. I wanted her to come with me because I did not want to stay in cold Utah, but she wanted to stay.

I miss my cowgirl who helped me get through cold winter nights. She was my American bush girl. I enjoy the memories we made though and have never forgotten her.

THE GYM, MY PLAYGROUND

The indoor gym, which is corporate, owned, is not the same as the natural outdoor world. It is a controlled environment, where you have to pay for a membership. There are security cameras everywhere, so it does not feel free. Most of the time, it is crowded, and whenever I went, I made sure to go and workout at a time when the gym is empty to avoid the heavy crowd. Generally, the music sucks, the place stinks, and the management does not care. Money is their only concern. The bathrooms are filthy because the members treat it as their personal mess hole.

They shit all over the toilet and do not even wash their hands before using the equipment. Most of the people there, men and women, have so many tattoos that their natural body is mutilated. It's also full of people juiced up with steroids, so their bodies are corrupted even more. It is sometimes impossible to know the difference between the male and female members, so it is best to keep your mouth shut before you end up labeling someone the wrong gender. Ha, who wants politics in the gym?

Honestly, people there will also steal every little thing they see, while others talk so much they are a distraction from exercise.

Going to the gym is like going to a human zoo in that you will see all kinds of strange phenomena. It's funny to see people with huge bellies and big muscles. They don't see the proportionality of their body, and they think they are body builders. I've seen people with tiny legs but gigantic arms. They look like they could tip over at any minute, and they walk with a disorganized sway to balance their cartoonish body shape. There are always the men who only work out their glam muscles, and they spend more time flexing in front of the mirror than actually working out. There are also always the tiny men who scream as they lift twenty pounds. You would think they were lifting up the moon.

Some pretty women there only want attention. They wear almost nothing, and they do sexual poses in front of everyone, but they never seem to work out. I am a man who finds women attractive, so this can be a bit distracting. It can be nice at times because it gives me a mental break and raises my testosterone level, but in the end, it just adds to an already chaotic environment.

Often, there is always tension or friction because people fight over little things, and the trainers do not help. Furthermore, dumb fat trainers and managers constantly harass people to buy or extend their membership. They also do not really teach their clients anything, for otherwise, their clients would not need them. Because the trainers are there for money, they have no incentive to make healthy, independent clients. Management also tells the trainers to mislead and only to show their clients enough progress to keep them happy, but not enough progress so that the member feels confident enough to work out on their own, away from the gym. The trainers give a constant stream of bad advice.

Most people only focus on losing weight, and trainers feed this fantasy, but I know better. When you lose weight, you lose muscle, and you may end up with sagging skin. I wanted to lose belly fat, build muscle, and get in shape. I decided to mix up my cardio training with some weight training to have a strong body. Losing muscle is no way to help or heal the body, and my mind began to understand this. In the end though, the gym is a worthy investment because the positives outweigh the negatives, and the gym has equipment for all types of people.

My genetic profile is that I am built like a runner. I am tall with a long body. Everybody has a different genetic makeup, and I was not at the gym to force my body into the shape of a body builder. I did not expect quick physical changes because real change takes time.

Going to the indoor gym and getting in shape is a boring process. I told my mind that patience is necessary, so I decided to be there five days a week as well. I use proper techniques, lots of repetition, and the isolation of my muscles to get in shape. I work out a different body part every thirty minutes. I believe in a total body workout. I follow my plan. I don't obsess, and I developed a system of weight lifting that worked for me and my goals.

When it comes to getting in shape, you can't copy what other people do. You have to work with your genetic makeup and develop a regiment that works for you specifically. You also need to commit by eating healthy foods most of the time.

Part of that commitment is that I don't talk with anyone at the gym. I keep to myself and focus on weight training. I see lots of people sitting around with their cell phones and talking away the time. Why come to the gym? Just to say they did, I suppose.

There are also those who scream, talk loud, and cuss to motivate themselves. It looks like a human zoo with all the animals in the same room. I just ignore it all as best I can, and I take my time to work out and think positive. The mind reminds the body that this is going to help me look good, feel good, and live a long healthy life.

Walking, jogging, running, lifting weights also made me tired. As a result, it made me sleep long good hours. After all, when you lift weights, you damage and tear muscles. The muscle strands then heal and are stronger than before. Sleeping is very important in this recovery process. Without the proper sleep, you will not see real physical, mental, spiritual, and soul improvements. Working out, though, usually leads to a better, deeper sleep, which refreshes the mind and rebuilds the body.

You do not need fancy shoes and new clothes to be at the gym. All you need is the will power and the discipline to workout. In that sense, it can be a very positive experience. I like being at the gym for many reasons. One of which is learning from others simply by observing. There are free lessons to be had, if I am willing to pay attention.

You can learn from everyone, including the old, the young, the disabled, and the many other characters the gym may bring. Those who are disabled, injured, and elderly impress me the most. They refuse to let any circumstances hold them back. Their will power to be there is motivating, and the innovations they use to stay healthy and in shape are inspiring. It gives me a different perspective on my own life and reminds me there are no excuses to let myself go. There are few places as open as the gym in the sense that just about any different type of person can come in and work out.

The gym generally promotes a friendly and inclusive environment, for every serious person there recognizes a kindred spirit in the journey to health. Serious conflict is rare, and people do not allow small things to affect and ruin the environment. In that sense, it can be a safe haven from the outside bullshit people allow to infect their minds.

Once I get to the gym and workout, my positive energy goes up and my troubles melt away. Negative voices desert my mind, and I feel as if I am starting fresh. My personality becomes infectious, and my mind, body, and soul's strength builds.

My confidence and mental awareness grows beyond believe. My flexibility, agility, posture, and balance improve. There are many free classes offered such as yoga, pilates, aerobics, martial arts, and many others. My overall conditioning improves, I feel the power of the universe running through my body, and I am truly conscious. Exercise, in that sense, brings with it the feeling of peace similar to that of religion.

YOU ARE NOT WHAT YOU EAT

You are not what you eat, and it is not all in the diet as others may claim. Most people are not genetically born fat, even though some people have diseases or conditions that make them retain weight. Most people blame their weight gain on their eating habits, parents, fast foods, schools, the government, and everything else they can point their finger. It's more of a mental issue than a physical one, and no one is to blame for the choices you make. Honestly, many people eat to become fat because there is a void in their lives.

Even though food is for the repairing, the growth, and the recovery of our bodies, most people eat food for comfort, taste, and smell. Social media and the moneymaking food industry play a big role in making us love food. Most people are tied to their foods emotionally, and it gives them the illusion of escaping the reality of life.

The taste distracts them from whatever is bothering them, so they feel at peace for a fleeting moment. Some people eat because they are always psychologically hungry. The body's only response is to turn a craving on to try and fix the issue, and their brain hungry pulse activates a switch.

People love sugar because it has pumped into their brains since conception. The food does not come to you, but rather, you go after the food. The food and drug lords spend billions of dollars to fuck with your head and make money. The people who buy these foods give them profits.

Understanding their dirty tactics has worked for me and helped me to break free of the mind tricks of the food industry. Teaching oneself and practicing discipline is the best way to control any weight gain, and it is the gateway to your weight loss. I am not disciplined every time, but most of the time, I am. I trick my mind and give it some of those foods it craves. I do not stress staying disciplined every second of every day. I take it easy and control my eating emotions. It is a learning process where you are constantly finding what you need to change in order for you to be healthy.

Another important way to monitor my weight gain is that I bought two different scales from different companies. Some scales can be off and mislead you. I weigh myself everyday whenever I want, and I do not stress about it. Total body weight is more important to me than counting calories. I do not use other forms of weight measurements.

I use simple addition and subtraction from the results of the scale. I know exactly how much weight I need to add or take off from my current total weight to stay healthy. The scale is my best friend because it tells me the truth. Being realistic and knowing exactly how much I weigh gives me the mind-set and the plan of action as far as exercise and eating habits are concerned.

I do not get emotional about gaining or losing weight because emotions fade away. Emotions thus are never a good motivation to improve. They will desert you before you make any real progress. This is why so many give up when they are just getting started. They make an emotional decision, and the desire burns out as soon as a proper distraction comes along.

Becoming healthy and fit should, to put it simply, be a logical decision. Honestly, how is that not the logical choice? What carries me through the long process of slow improvement is staying disciplined most of the time and allowing myself to eat junk foods here or there. However, the whole time I eat these junk foods; it feeds my craving for dysfunction. These moments satisfy the need to occasionally stray from the path. It feels good to break the rules, and it provides some extra motivation the next time I work out.

The fact that I feel terrible physically after eating junk is extra motivation because it proves my body does not want it. It is an effective reminder of just how bad this garbage food is for me. It is like a vacation from a job, I know I will be back to work soon. Part of the logic in this is knowing exactly what I need to do to get back on track.

Some people might be saying that they cannot stray from the path or slip up occasionally. They argue that if they give in a little, then their behavior will snow ball out of control, and they will fall back into unhealthy habits. This is the wrong mind-set to have. It is an excuse for failure because you have already decided you have absolutely no self-control, so you must be strict all the time. This is not solving the problem though, for it is merely avoiding your problems. An approach sets-up failure.

Losing weight is not always the right approach to getting healthy. When you lose weight, you also lose muscle mass and end up with saggy skin.

Some people do not need to lose weight, and they only need strengthen their body and gain muscle, which will actually make them gain weight. This, however, is good weight gain.

Besides running and lifting weights, I fast most of the nights until the middle of the following day. I jog and run without eating any food and simply drink water. This method burns the visceral fat from all its hiding places in my body. The fasting clears my mind and allows my brain to use real energy stored from the foods I ate the day before. When you sleep, your body converts excess sugar to glucose. This means that it will no longer be the primary source of energy for the next day. Eventually, the glucose converts to glycogen, which is an energy reserve that your body rarely accesses.

The body cells do not know what to do with it, and it becomes a permanent store. This is the visible fat on people, so I fast because it calms me down, and it is the best combination I found: running, jogging, resting, and fasting. As a result, my body has no chance to store excess energy sources. I only eat two meals a day and those two meals provide plenty of calories for my body to operate without going into excess

RUNNING WITH WHITE PEOPLE

As a professor, I walked home like everyone else. There were many people walking to their cars. I never felt any fear or danger among the students that were walking to their cars. I have done this many years, and have never had any moments of scariness or violence. I walked through the dark streets that led to my house, never afraid.

My students would always say, "Aren't you afraid someone will attack you or harm you?" And my response was, "No, I don't think of any of that." I never felt alone because I believe that there is always a Higher Power watching over me, so I do not feel afraid.

Instead, I enjoy walking through the nice night's cool breeze because it reminds me of walking through the bushes of Jamama Town.

One night was different. I was walking home, and there was a bunch of white people walking about twenty feet in front of me. They were going to the parking lot. I was wearing all black. All of a sudden, I heard a loud noise coming from the white people in front of me.

A white person said, "Jennifer, run, run, let's run. He's coming..." They repeated this many times, and I freaked out.

I started running behind them. I said to myself that whatever these white people were running from, I had better run from it too.

I was not going to be left alone with who or whatever they were running from. It is also human nature to run when you see other people suddenly run, especially a large group. I took off after them, and with my long legs, I started to catch up.

"Run. He is coming. He is coming. Run. He is coming. Run."

The faster they ran, the faster I ran because I did not want to be alone with the danger they were running from. They got into their cars, and slammed the doors. They started their engines and said, "Here he is," and sped off.

I looked back and realized that they were running from me the whole time. I started flipping them off and yelling at them as they sped off saying, "Racist bitches." I was having a hard time walking because I was so angry about their social phobia. I did not learn of this type of phobia until that night. I had not realized how scared some white people are of black people,

Some people are scared of others simply because of the stereotypes that pervade society. Fear of others is something we are not born with; it is something we learn. It is like a disease that causes panic, stress, and sometimes violence. The fear spreads to those around the infected, and the cycle continues. Walking home, I did not feel the pleasantness of the cool breeze. My anger was too great in that moment. I would not change anything about that day though. If I see people yelling, screaming, and running, I would still take off. Looking back, it is kind of fun, and I laugh about the situation.

WAKE UP AMERICA

There is a system and a society no matter where you live. The system consists of groups of people who are committed to their ideology, which is to lie, exploit, murder, assassinate, and dumb-down society. They have strong social media that deceive, distort, and flood the brains of society with fake news.

It is all about making money because money creates power and power creates control. Don't be fooled. Everything is controlled by the system including your personal information.

The banks control the systems. Without money, the systems will not function. Taxation of the society creates infinite amount of wealth that fill up the banks' coffers along with their front, the government.

The banks and the system are partners in crime. It's all about business. The banks loan money to the system to establish military, police, corporations, politicians, educational systems, pharmaceutical companies, food industry, justice departments, Secret societies, prisons, presidents and politicians, International organizations, hospitals, sports and entertainment industries.

Every system in the world wants to have the best technological, military, and nuclear power to control the ebb and flow of the earth. The world itself is shaped in a way that allows world powers to exploit poorer and weaker governments. People often fail to acknowledge that the 3rd world was established and is perpetuated by dominant nations to maintain their positions of control and wealth.

The Far East Asians and the Russians are on the hunt to take over the entire planet for global domination. The Middle East are fighting among themselves for religious reasons, while their oil is being pumped through the Mediterranean and boosting foreign powers. Every nation oppresses their society to hang on power, and everyone has had their own form of slavery. Slavery is business.

The African tribal chiefs sold their own people to the white system for money. Slavery is inhuman and deplorable. The rest of the world watched and benefitted as Africans were lynched, murdered, raped, whipped, spit on, despised, and their rights were denied. How can you blame the Europeans for colonizing and enslaving Africans when our own leaders are so corrupted that they sell their own people?

I grew up in a tribal system where a few tribes dominate all the other tribes. They murder, rape, burn properties, and imprison others and make them eat their own shit. They beat my mother, killed some of my relatives, friends, and tied them behind their trucks and dragged them on the streets until their entire bodies broke and shred apart. These vicious murderers are people that we knew our whole lives, who lived with us in the villages, and they can turn around whenever they want and harm whomever they choose.

These same people commit atrocities and claim that we believe in the same God and the same religion. These are the descendants of the tribal chiefs who sold our people to slavery under the whites, Arabs, Persians, and the Jews. They allowed European colonials to exploit Africa and colonize our land so that they could boost their own wealth and power.

The United States took the European model, and their cultural hierarchy is now a model for the world. It began with the new royalty, the slave and landowners, and robber barons. However, once open slavery was no longer publicly accepted, they established a new underclass: pitting freed slaves against poor whites for economic survival. This "white trash" class is disgruntled and unfulfilled, but has a strongly built cultural patriotism.

They see an escape and glory in the military. The same military pillages foreign nations of their resources. At the same time, being given a purpose, they rarely see how they help contribute to the system that exploits them.

Culturally, a veil is pulled over their eyes, things become fuzzy, and those in power, (a tradition established by royalty, slave and landowners) give them plenty of scapegoats to be distracted by, whether blacks, immigrants, commies, etc. So fully brainwashed into the cultural order, the people easily find low income and simple work that keeps them exactly where those on top want them to be: angry at each other on the lower end of the economy.

The sons and daughters of slave owners (the new royalty) thus maintain the social arrangement by using the institutions of the country established by their ancestors. Churches and schools help to shape young minds as well as remind older generations of what they have been taught. TV , movies and social media recycle images that go back to the establishment of slavery.

These images help to perpetuate and reinforce stereotypes and old rivalries. Laws are balanced in favor of certain groups in the hierarchy and are used to continue divisions in the culture. The military helps to reinforce the concept of national superiority and cultural opposition.

This model of divide and conquer has helped to shape the world as it is today. Those in power establish fake oppositions to create rivalries that establish a subservient mentality.

Corporations, not society, own and mold the world. Follow the banks and you will find out what your own money is spent. Billions of dollars are spent on dumbing down and brainwashing human minds. The use of pesticides on the foods we eat promotes deadly diseases such as cancer, nerve disorders, and lower the immune system. The foods laced with pesticides are exported to the developing countries, feed their populations to keep them sick, keep them from growing their own foods, and spread many diseases.

These infested foods feed the cows and other animals we eat, and we drink their milk. Diseases such as obesity, mental illness, cancer, and major body organs are the result of mindlessly eating this food.

Meanwhile, major animal and plant species have disappeared and some are dying out every day. I see thousands of dead bees and birds every year from pesticides in our own environment.

The water we drink is no longer safe, so they build modern medical hospitals to keep us sick and force a dependency on modern medicine.

I don't use the word racism lightly because not everyone is a racist, and I only speak from my personal experience. I don't think it is fair for any ethnic or racial group to be labelled as racists. When you understand the difference between system and society, you will find out that most white Americans are not racist and have been unfairly labelled as such.

My first day in America at Cal Poly in San Luis Obispo, everywhere I looked, there were white people. I had never seen so many white people in all my life. Some were walking, some studying, some hanging out, some eating, and some playing music. One of the best ways I learn is by observing what other people do because I find that you can learn from everyone.

I saw some students sleeping on the green grass of the campus. At first, I thought they were homeless and did not have a place to live, but then, I realized they were just resting for their next class.

I was so tired that I fell asleep with a bunch of white people under the blue skies. I felt like I was in the village, where I would sleep in the open environment. It was comforting to find that not everything in America was different.

San Luis Obispo is the best place that I have ever lived. It is a place that I grew up mentally, and I was welcomed and treated wonderfully. I played music in coffee houses, public libraries, and on the streets. I never felt any racism, nor was I racially profiled or discriminated against. I travelled with students on field trips and learned more about the area.

The acceptance and openness of others allowed me to open my mind and kept me from locking out others. As a result, I was better able to integrate and to see the world with a more flexible point of view. It was an awesome experience to connect with a new community in such a way and to see an appreciation of difference.

People are at peace, health oriented, and very kind. If I can turn back the clock, I should have never left San Luis Obispo.

I didn't know much about American history or culture. All I had heard was that all white people were rich. Literally, people spoke as if money was everywhere. I realize now that this is not true, and I understand there are white people who are poor or homeless. The physical proof was in front of me every time I walked around the city. People struggling to get by became the evidence of America's poverty.

When I moved to Utah, the culture was a little different in that the majority were Mormons, but their treatment of me did not change. They were open and curious, and it was very easy to interact with the people there. In that regard, nothing changed, and I was able to adjust easily.

You do not know anything about racial profiling unless you have been stopped, searched, beaten, jailed, imprisoned, or even murdered. The cops who racially profile are not only white, but brainwashed other ethnic Americans

The truth is that the issue is not about good cops or bad cops; that mentality is a distraction. The system is the problem and until it's changed, oppression will continue. Racial profiling is ingrained into the American justice system

The first time I experienced racism was in Riverside, California, where I worked as a professor. I was hired to teach Health Science and Biology lecture and labs. I was the only black person that the Department of Science had ever offered a job. I could sense a strange tension or hostility. The faculty looked white, but they were not like the friendly white people that I had met in San Luis Obispo and Utah. To me, this was a different breed of whites with a different mentality.

When I started at the college, they allowed me to teach Health lecture and Biology lab, but they did not allow me to teach Biology lecture. This was my first assignment as a professor, and I wondered why I was not allowed to teach Biology lecture when all the other new (white) professors were allowed to teach whatever class they wanted. I have a PhD in Biological Sciences, while the others did not.

They supervised me at all times. They wanted me to abandon my teaching style and adapt to their way of teaching. I was never going to do that. I gravitated towards my teaching style, which 95% of the students loved. It was a combination of subject matter, laughter, discussions, and interactions. I also enjoyed this free style of teaching. My way of teaching did not sit well with the whites in charge.

The hiring process is one of the phoniest processes at the college level, and human resources control it. It is all a matter of who you know and their connections. Ninety percent of the people working at the college know each other or have known each other. A small percentage of professors get hired on by luck and desperation on the part of the university.

They put out fliers of information on the college websites and newspapers. They list the requirements for hiring. These are all lies because they already know who they want to hire.

I know so because I, as a professor, was on the hiring committee

There were a whole family of brothers, sisters, mothers, and fathers all working at the college. The system is rigged against strong minds, and the college is bloated with academic incest.

Even in black Africa, I suffered tribal discrimination because my father's tribe is so black that they glow in the dark. I was never treated fairly because my father's tribe is considered minority because of their skin color and their number.

I never received any favoritism or privilege in Somalia or America. I earned all my success. I succeeded in America, and from my personal experience, most Americans are not racist.

Racism, tribalism, and discrimination will never go away. It is part of the system of any country. The system is going to stay because societies are weakened and mentally controlled. They can protest all they want. They can scream and demonstrate, but they will not cause any changes. Not really. The system will only create the illusion of change. All the movements, which are anti-this, anti-that are fake. They are created and funded by the system to keep society confused, in conflict, chaotic, and chasing imaginary foes.

TAKE A SHIT

I believe unconventional way is the best method one can learn and stay focused. I was often criticized for how I presented my lessons. As long as the students learn and retain the material, the method should not matter. I would try to get creative because I am teaching some really dry information to students who are not science majors. However, the institution would rather I just stand and read from a textbook rather than teach an unorthodox lesson on a subject like "fiber" in Health class.

One of the most important foods is fiber. As a professor who teaches about health and nutrition, I always put an emphasis on eating foods that contain fiber. This is a basic health fact, and it is to the benefit of my students. On the other hand, I am not a big fan of how the book teaches the subject because they get too technical, and there is nothing attached to the information to help students remember or relate to the material.

The textbook uses big ass words to explain the word cellulose, a polysaccharide that is found in plant cell walls that we are unable to digest because we don't have the proper enzymes to break it down.

The way that I simplify it to my students is by explaining that cellulose is fiber material. I then attach a story or information to it to help the students remember it. Something that I always tell my students as part of this lesson is that there is a relationship between the attitude of human beings and their shit. People who take a shit at least once a day are happier than the ones who don't.

I explain to the students that if they go home or see their friends during the day, you can tell the ones who took a shit from the ones who did not. The ones who didn't take a shit look stressed, grumpy, and angry. If you were to ask them if they took a shit, then they would say, "no." I explain that those who say," yes," seem happier and more playful, and sometimes even sing because the load of toxic shit has come out of their body. It makes a person feel lighter, and the blood flows better through the body.

The lungs are able to breath better, and the heart is not as congested, so it is better able to pump fresh oxygenated blood throughout the body, as well as send fresh nutrients to the cells throughout the body. I emphasize this point by explaining that corn is a food that can't be digested completely because we don't have the enzymes for it to digest, so some of the corn comes out of our body. Therefore, when you see corn in your shit, that usually means you're healthy. It also means that most of the toxins have been cleaned out from your body.

Once the toxins are removed from your intestinal tract, the toxins of your mind will also be eliminated. It ties together because I explain to students that they need to eat their corn because it doesn't cost much, and you will have a lot of fiber, which is good for you. You will be happy that you did. When you see your friends and family members are grumpy and stressed, ask if they have taken a shit today.

I would tell my students that I had literally and figuratively walked through shit in my life. In the world, some people would shit in the bushes, and you might step in it sometimes. However, it was clear to you who ate corn the night before. I'd think, "Damn, my uncle took a shit last night. At least he's eating his corn." This would get a laugh out of students, and they'd remember this story.

My job is to primarily instruct freshman, and to break down information that is more complicated in order to make it easier to absorb. Not all of my students are science majors, and not all of them care about this information. As a professor who wants all of his students to learn, I have to re-heat it into something they can digest. I guarantee they won't have trouble remembering what cellulose is and what it is for. The students laugh during the lesson, and remember it because it keeps their attention. This is far more effective than bombarding them with big words they won't remember. It also helps put personal health into perspective for them.

I explain to students that, when it comes to eating, it is ok to have a fuck up day during the week. That means you can eat or drink and junk-food or garbage they want. We can't be good all the time. At the same time, I phrase it as "fuck-up day" because it's ok to fuck up once in a while, but it's not ok to fuck up every day.

This type of phrasing helps them remember this fact, and the openness leaves them more open to approaching a healthier life-style.

Sometimes, I run into some students at anywhere. I didn't see them in a long time, and suddenly they bring up the "shitting in the bushes story." It was funny and random, but the story clearly works. Interestingly, they said they could remember it because they could relate to the ridiculousness of it.

WHY I STAY LOOKING GOOD

Cardio and weight lifting exercises have become part of my life. I developed a soul of patience and planned to take my time and learn from my mistakes. I relax and enjoy every day that I am out there exercising.

The lemon water that I drink boosts my immune system, cleanses my body, and leads to better circulation and efficient nutrient absorption. The rays from the ninety-three million miles of sunlight drain the toxins out of my body and make my skin glisten and shine with sweat. Vitamin D is a gift from the sun. With the summer heat, the melanin flows to the surface of my skin and makes me look like a black diamond on the road.

I have developed a habit of taking hot and cold showers. The cold water running over my body reminds me of when I used to swim in the Juba River as a child in Jamama Town. I always had a fear of the cold water because it made me take a deep breath as I plunged into it. Swimming was the only way to cool off while growing up in a world without air conditioning. This gave me motivation to overcome the fear of cold water, and I improved my breathing process as a natural side effect. Now, I tend to be more alert and awake. This state is enhanced by the food I eat.

My diet consists mostly of plant-based foods, but I also eat small amounts of chicken, fish, raw eggs, and occasionally, fast foods. Some of these foods contain proteins, carbohydrates, fats, and fiber. Over time, my metabolism improved, and my enzymes break foods down faster. The chicken and the fish contain complete proteins, which are broken down into amino acids. The amino acids are easily absorbed through the blood stream and get into my cells faster. This complicated process requires time, so it keeps the metabolism active longer. I eat plenty of plant materials. Typically, I eat a mixture of beans and rice to convert incomplete proteins into complete proteins. Complete proteins are proteins that contain the most important amino acids. My body cannot produce these integral amino acids, so I eat chicken and fish. Proteins consist of Carbon, Hydrogen, Oxygen, and Nitrogen. All of which are natural elements that our bodies need to be healthy and fit.

I have noticed that, along with the exercise, lifting weights, eating proteins, and getting proper rest allowed me to gain more muscle. Getting enough rest also allowed my bones, ligaments, and cartilage to strengthen. In addition, my immune system and antibodies increased and more efficiently protect my body from diseases. Furthermore, by eating proteins, my hemoglobin's oxygen carrying capacity improved, so now fresh oxygen gets to my cells faster, and I can breathe better. This allowed me to improve my lung capacity, and I am able to jog faster while covering longer distances. This is a natural and lengthy process of improvement.

I don't take any protein supplements or any steroids to enhance my workouts and build muscle. Those sorts of supplements pollute the body and corrupt its natural abilities. I take supplements like iron, potassium, magnesium, fish oil, and calcium pills. These are the natural ingredients to improvement. I am comfortable eating natural foods and put the work in no matter how long it takes. As long as I see small increments of progress, I know I am on the right track. I am not competing with anyone else, and I understand my genetic profile. It is important for people to know that there are no easy, one trick solutions to getting in shape. A person either wants it enough to do the work, or they don't, but putting in the work doesn't have to mean being completely strict in your habits.

Yes, I eat junk and fast foods. They taste good, and I have to trick my mind to overcome the cultural brainwashing of the food industry. The fact is we are all inundated with food industry ads. These have us craving certain foods we know we do not need, so it is ok to trick that craving into thinking it is being satisfied. At the same time, I eat junk food occasionally, and it should not be a daily or even weekly habit.

I feel great, look good, and I actually see the transformation of my body strength. My belly fat melted away, and my arms and shoulders look bigger. In addition, my skin looks healthier and my legs and heart muscle got stronger. They carry me so much better through all the running, and my heart no longer chokes when strained.

Sadly, it's human nature for people to judge others by their looks. This is inevitable, but what people discover as they make progress is that others will begin to acknowledge that progress. Comments like, "You look good," or, "Have you been working out," suddenly come.

This builds confidence and motivation. The outlook on the world is different, and the aura around you will become lighter and more magnetic. It's like a positivity wave that gathers more and more energy and keeps riding up the coast without crashing. This will cause you to feel a new status, and you will walk a little taller. Women will notice too. Suddenly, they'll be touching your arms or your shoulder here or there. It's funny because it's like a cute puppy walked in, and they just have to pet it. Only, you aren't a puppy.

The ladies everywhere are buzzing around me, and I roar among them like the lion from the African savannah, not like the lion from the American zoo.

BAD SEX

There is a lot of pressure on the minds of students sitting in a boring classroom. Some students have a long day of work, some don't like to be there because most of the teachers are boring, and some don't like it because the educational system is so fucked up. I have been a student all my life, so I perfectly understand what it is like to be in their situation.

Students looked forward to my classes every day because they knew I would turn their bad days into positive, shining ones. They would forget their troubles because of the laughter and positive energy I would bring to them. I created a positive environment in which almost everybody felt comfortable and interacted with each other. I turned my teaching into healing sessions.

I used humor as a technique to bond with students because it is the most powerful tool to heal the human soul, and laughter is the best way to capture student's interest. I incorporate comedic stories into my teaching because it makes the students interact and laugh, for science class, in my experience, can be boring.

One day, I was teaching a chapter about stress, and somehow, I started the class by asking the students what stresses them most. The responses were typical causes such as bills, traffic, family, and relationships. Suddenly and unexpectedly, one woman said she was stressed because her boyfriend had a small dick, and he couldn't satisfy her.

The class erupted into laughter, and within a few seconds, the entire class came to life. Another student quickly responded to her by saying she must have a loose vagina, so she needs a "pussy glue" to hold it all together. He also said she should tighten up her pussy by doing keggles, which is an exercise that strengthens the vaginal walls. A female student agreed with him and said her own pussy is loose because she uses big sex toys and finds men with big dicks. The whole class burst in laughter again and got so excited about the subject matter.

It's raunchy, but it is something young students can relate to because it is on their minds. People are too sensitive, so students tend to be quiet in class to avoid upsetting others, but once they hear things like this, they loosen up (pun intended), and they feel like they can be themselves.

As a professor, I found the discussions exciting and hilarious because of the random shit that comes out of students' mouths.

One time, a lady in my class said she did not like the sex discussion because she is religious, and it bothered her. One male student responded that he is very religious and loves the class discussion because he never heard such crazy sex stories. He continued by explaining that when he got home, he was going to masturbate, and the class started to laugh more. Another said he likes to listen the sounds of his girlfriend's pussy because it gets him more excited.

The discussion went on, so many started to participate, and I had no idea that so many human beings are such super freaks. A lady told the class that she never allows her boyfriend to have sex with her unless he licks all over her body including her butt hole, and someone said that is "disgusting and weak," but she said she didn't care because that was what she wanted, and if he could not perform, she'd kick him to the curb. Some of the men and women were into threesomes, all combinations of them.

Almost everyone was thrown off when one guy told the class that the best stress relief is when he pisses on his girlfriend's head, drinks his urine, and then, she shits on his head. Someone else said she would tie up, blindfold, and whip their partner. Another student said he would hang his girlfriend from chains, tie her on the cross, and fuck her.

Someone said that he could not stand pussy that stinks like dead fish, and the way to tell them that their pussy stinks by putting his finger in it, and put it to their nose, so they can catch the dead fish stank. Story after story came (pun intended again) out, and you can guarantee students remembered that day's lesson.

Now, before anyone gets his or her panties in a wad about this being a college classroom, it is important to keep in mind that I taught health science. Sex and STD's are a part of the curriculum. However, just lecturing from a textbook is boring, and no students care. If I weave lessons in and around humorous discussions though, the students often found the lessons easier to remember. I do not start these discussions. They just happen spontaneously, and I enjoy listening to an unscripted lesson plan that brings lots of fun in the class. Humor eases the tension and the negative stress. If students remember the material because of the strange story they heard that day, then the job is accomplished.

SAN LUIS OBISPO

I thought when I came to America I'd be leaving music behind, but when I got to San Luis Obispo, I realized that was not the case. During the first week I spent in America, I did a lot of walking. As I walked around downtown, I was surrounded by music. I followed the sounds of the drums. They pulled me to them. The heart, to me, is a drum, and the sound of that beat called to it. It led me to a nice little place called The Mission Inn Creek. It is a beautiful creek surrounded by nice restaurants.

As I approached the sounds, I saw people of different colors drumming together. Where I was from, I was used to people of the same color drumming together. However, this drum circle had variety; it even white people with dread locks. This caught me off guard because they were playing beats that I had heard back home.

A strange epiphany washed over me in that moment and it set my heart on fire. I felt like a celestial being, as though my ancestors visited me in this moment. A spiritual energy surrounded and moved through me, and I saw the way that music connects people. I wanted to join in so badly, despite the fact that they were strangers. The circle of drums carried me home for a moment, and I ached for that connection.

Finally, I could no longer contain myself, and using my broken English, and rudimentary sign language, I asked to join their drum circle. Music doesn't know a language, so all the leader of the circle wanted to know is, "Can you play?" I motioned yes, and he handed me a djembe, so I became a part of the drum circle. It was a little multi-cultural community, and as diverse as we all were, we began conversing in music, and that's because music has its own language and a unified spirit. They were surprised at how well I could play, and they asked me to come to their circle again. After that, I went there once or twice a week. I asked them where I could get a guitar.

They pointed me to a nearby store, and I bought my first guitar. I used some of my scholarship money, and it was well spent. The first time I played the guitar just felt right.

I didn't need any sheet music or training; it came fairly naturally. I was playing blues notes and rhythms from Somali music. Everybody thinks that I went to school and studied how to play musical instruments. I actually just seem to play naturally with no instruction needed. I never use a metronome to feel the beat; it is already built in me. My heart beat is my metronome. I stuck with that drum circle, and worked on my guitar skills throughout the rest of my time in San Luis Obispo.

One of the hardest things about leaving there was leaving that drum circle. They were a good bunch of people, and we had a deep connection through music. However, when my visa was running out, I knew I had to leave. It was a hard choice to make, but I knew that even if the people changed, I could bring the music with me, and that's what I did when I went to Utah.

I still get teary eyes when I think of the people of San Luis Obispo. The most important lesson they left me with was that good, loving people are found among people of every color and ethnic group. For me, this was a tremendous and uplifting experience to find so many good people in one place who did not care about color or creed, and this could not have been a better situation for my first years in America.

PERCEPTION IS NOT A REALITY

Perception only becomes a reality if you believe it, and another's view can infect your perception if you believe the delusional mind-sets of haters. You don't have to prove anything to anyone, and all you have to do is keep believing in yourself. Growing up, I was told I was too dumb to accomplish anything. I always knew I was better than most of the people labelling me because I believed in myself. The haters already determined my future, but they had no idea the power of mind and the strength of my spirit, which resided within me.

I never tried to prove anything to anyone but myself, and I always kept to myself because my thoughts were all I cared about. Haters kept bragging, judging me, and predicting my future of failures, but I knew something they didn't know, which is that life is like a marathon, and it's not over until you cross the finish line. The label "dumb" did not bother me because the more they talked, the more energy they wasted, and the more I prepared myself for success.

We did not have any libraries, but I still read books and worked on my math and science skills. Out of thousands of students from my home country, I earned a scholarship to the Somali University. I also earned a scholarship to Cal Poly San Luis Obispo of the United States of America for a master's degree in sciences. In less than two years, I completed my master's degree and was accepted at Utah State University, where I completed my PhD in biological sciences. Shortly after I earned my PhD, I was hired as a professor in a college in Southern California.

I write and publish my own books and found out that I have unique way of writing and expressing my opinions. I am born with the talent of playing music, and I produce my own music. I inspired thousands of students through my music, teaching, and my books.

Nothing replaces hard work and believing in yourself.

Don't be fooled. Most people on the planet don't care about your progress, so self-reliance is the way to success. Never give up no matter what.

Their realities and perceptions are not yours, and they are not mine. Everybody has a chance, but complacency and outside influences are the enemies of self-improvement and success. Don't let their words and thoughts infect your own. Move on forward.

KNOW YOUR HEART

Your life is dependent on oxygen, and without a healthy heart that properly pumps the oxygen through the body, you are in lots of trouble. In addition, your heart distributes nutrients, hormones, transmits neurological signals, and sends sexual feelings through the blood. In addition, you need healthy lungs that bring oxygen from outside your body to oxygenate the recycled blood, which has lots of carbon dioxide and other dirt particles in it.

I read and taught from many textbooks about the human heart, and it always seemed too complicated and too boring to understand. I always believed unconventional ways of teaching are the best ways for students to learn and stay focused.

I came up with a simple way you can learn the general function of the human heart without the big ass words. The human heart consists of four chambers, and let's just call them, for the sake of understanding, Rooms. The human heart consists of four Rooms:

Room#1 = Right atrium

Room#2 = Right ventricle

Room#3 = Left atrium

Room#4 = Left Ventricle

There is a valve in between each two Rooms and lets call them, for the sake of understanding, two windows.

Window #1 = Tricuspid valve

Window #2 = Bicuspid valve

The human heart is divided into two, the right and the left side. The right side of the heart pumps deoxygenated blood. The left side of the heart pumps oxygenated blood

Let us just say that, for the sake of learning, deoxygenated = bad blood (without oxygen) or blue blood even though there is no such a thing as blue blood despite how it looks. It only appears blue, but it simply has no oxygen, and it is full of the junk picked up throughout the body.

Yellow color in the heart or body = fat.

Oxygenated = good blood (with oxygen), or red blood, because it is full of oxygen.

A membrane called the septum doesn't allow the two bloods to mix and separates the two sides. The septum = bridge

BLOOD FLOW

1. Bad blood or deoxygenated is collected in room # 1

2. Then it goes through window #1 and is collected in room# 2

3. Window # 1 closes to prevent back blood flow.

4. Room #2 contracts and pushes the bad blood through pulmonary artery to the lungs

5. The lungs oxygenate the bad blood, and it turns red because of the oxygen you breathe in is added to it, so it becomes good blood. You breathe in oxygen and breathe out carbon dioxide.

6. Oxygenated or good blood returns into room # 3 from the lungs through the pulmonary vein.

7. Oxygenated blood or good blood Goes through window # 2

8. Good blood is collected in Room # 4

9. Window # 2 closes to prevent back blood flow.

10. Room # 4 contracts and pumps good blood into the aorta.

11. The aorta, the biggest pump, sends good blood across the body.

TAKING CARE OF YOUR HEART

Drink water

Walk, jog, run, bike, swim, and lift weights. Exercise regularly.

Don't stress the negative bullshit

Stop smoking and drinking

Watch your weight gain. Weigh yourself on daily basis

Change negative thoughts into positive thoughts

Don't hang out with the haters, the low lives, and the losers.

Shut the hell up and let your heart rest

Smile and laugh like you are a psycho

Listen to the music you like

Take a break and relax

Live in the present because you can't do anything about the past

When people say, "I love you from the bottom of my heart," they are really saying, "I love you from the bottom of my ventricles." The ventricles (room 2 and 4) contract and push the blood out, so they give to the rest of the body. No one ever says, "I love you from the top of my heart," which would be the atriums (Room 1 and 3).

That's because these only receive blood from the body. This is true when people say, "I feel you." It's because they feel the contraction of the heart, and how you make it react.

"Sexual healing" follows the same principle. The ventricles of the heart pump blood to the sex organs. Thus, it gets the whole body reacting. Sexual chemistry thus is rooted in the heart. The heart also helps purify and refresh the body, so sexual feelings boost this purification cycle, so they help us heal. It also makes us think less because when aroused, all the blood rushes to the genitals, which limits the brain's oxygen levels. Sexual feeling is at its peak at the moment of orgasm. People are at their dumbest in this moment, and this is one of the reasons they will say the most nonsensical things when busting their nuts.

Both good and evil thoughts travel through the blood and are pumped by the heart all over the body, so it affects every parts of our lives.

The heart and blood find their way symbolically into many aspects of culture. Even without realizing, the gangs called the Crips and Bloods incorporated this in their symbols. For they chose the colors blue and red to represent their differences.

The colors, of course, represent the two types of blood. Why choose this? Because there is discord, or bad blood, between them. In that sense, parts of our natural body always seem to find their way into our representations through speech and images.

People put a huge emphasis on family or "blood" relation. Blood is thicker than water, as the saying goes. The sharing of genetic material in the blood is a bond we instinctually sense. The heart controls the flow of the blood, so the two images together have always found their way into the cultural representations and lexicon we use. The heart's health is integral to survival, not just in the sense of avoiding a heart attack. Healthy blood flow affects weight gain, immune response, and the distribution of energy throughout the body. Without a healthy heart, all of these falter, and it leads to a downward spiral in our health.

Take care of your heart because heart attack is the number one killer in the world.

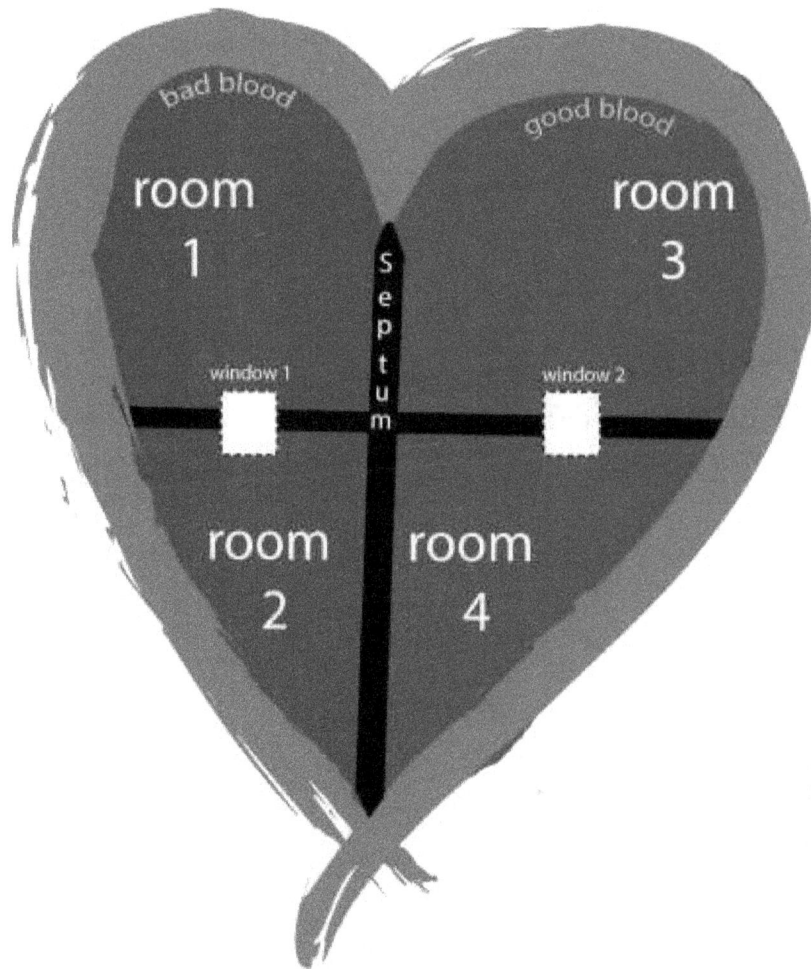

bad blood

good blood

room 1

room 3

septum

window 1

window 2

room 2

room 4

Check out the color version of the heart on the cover page of the book

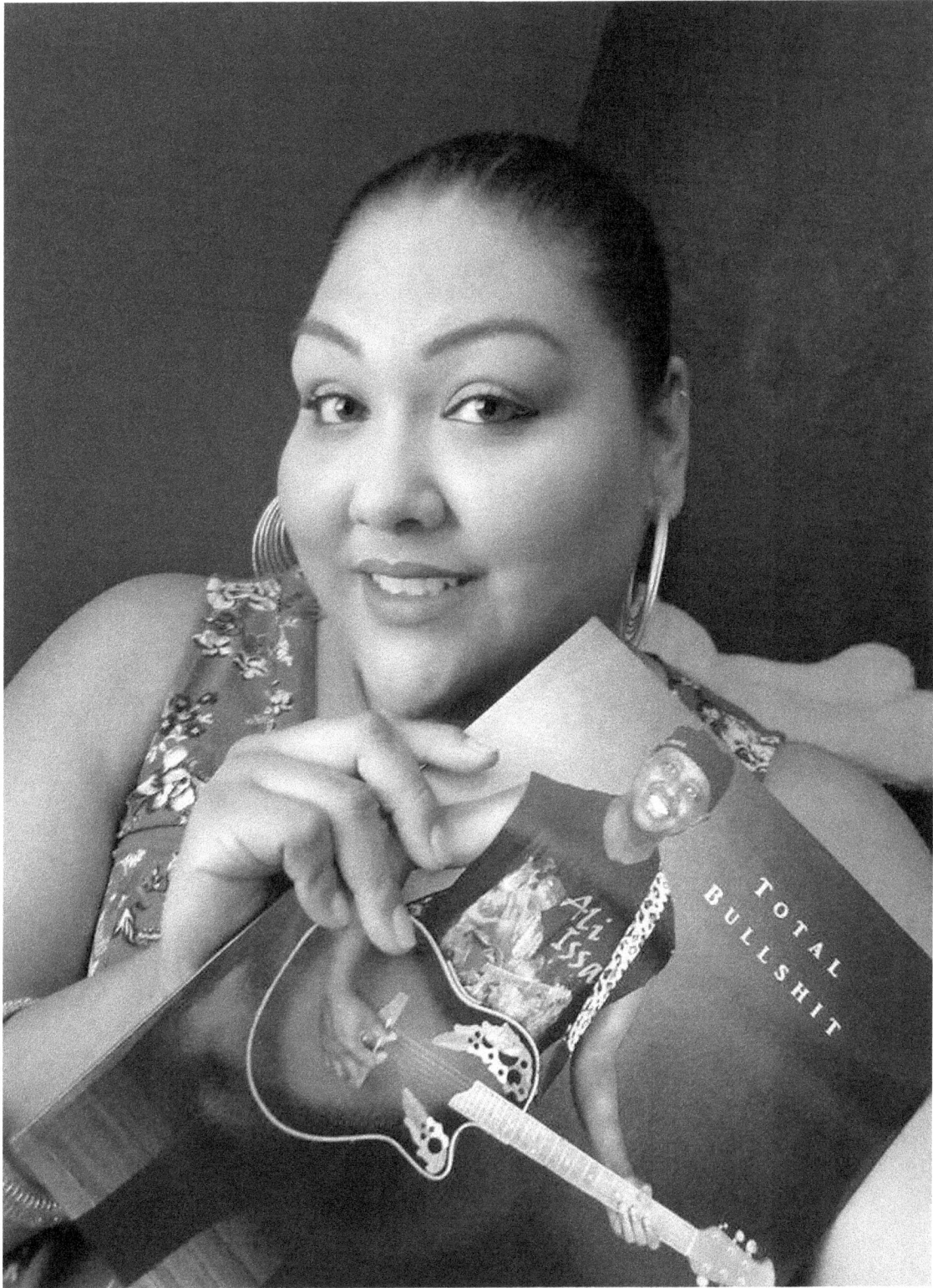

JULIA PUT MY FIRST BOOK ON THE WORLD STAGE.
SHE IS GENUINE, KIND
AND UNCONDITIONALLY SUPPORTIVE

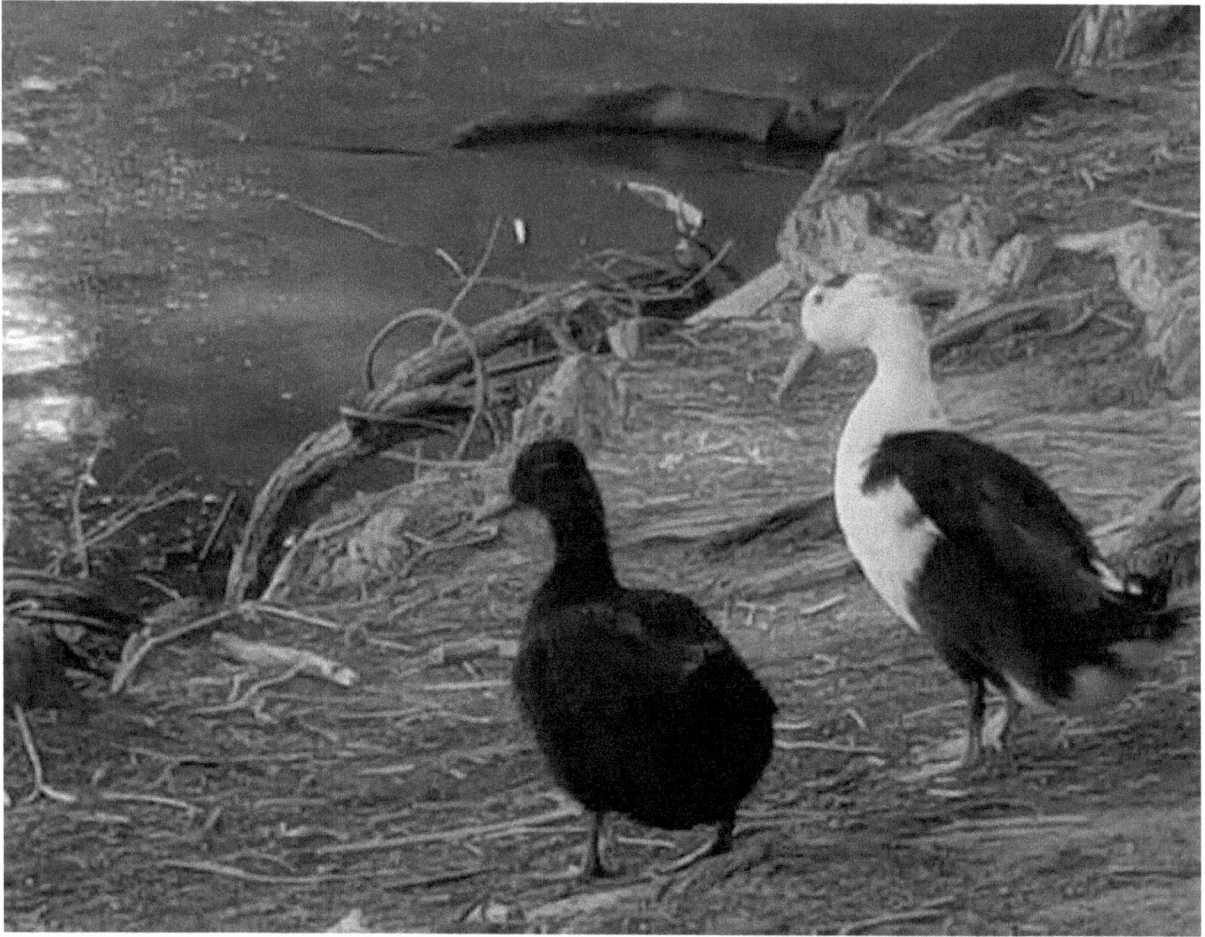

IT'S EASY TO GET ALONG
WHEN YOU ARE MENTALLY STRONG

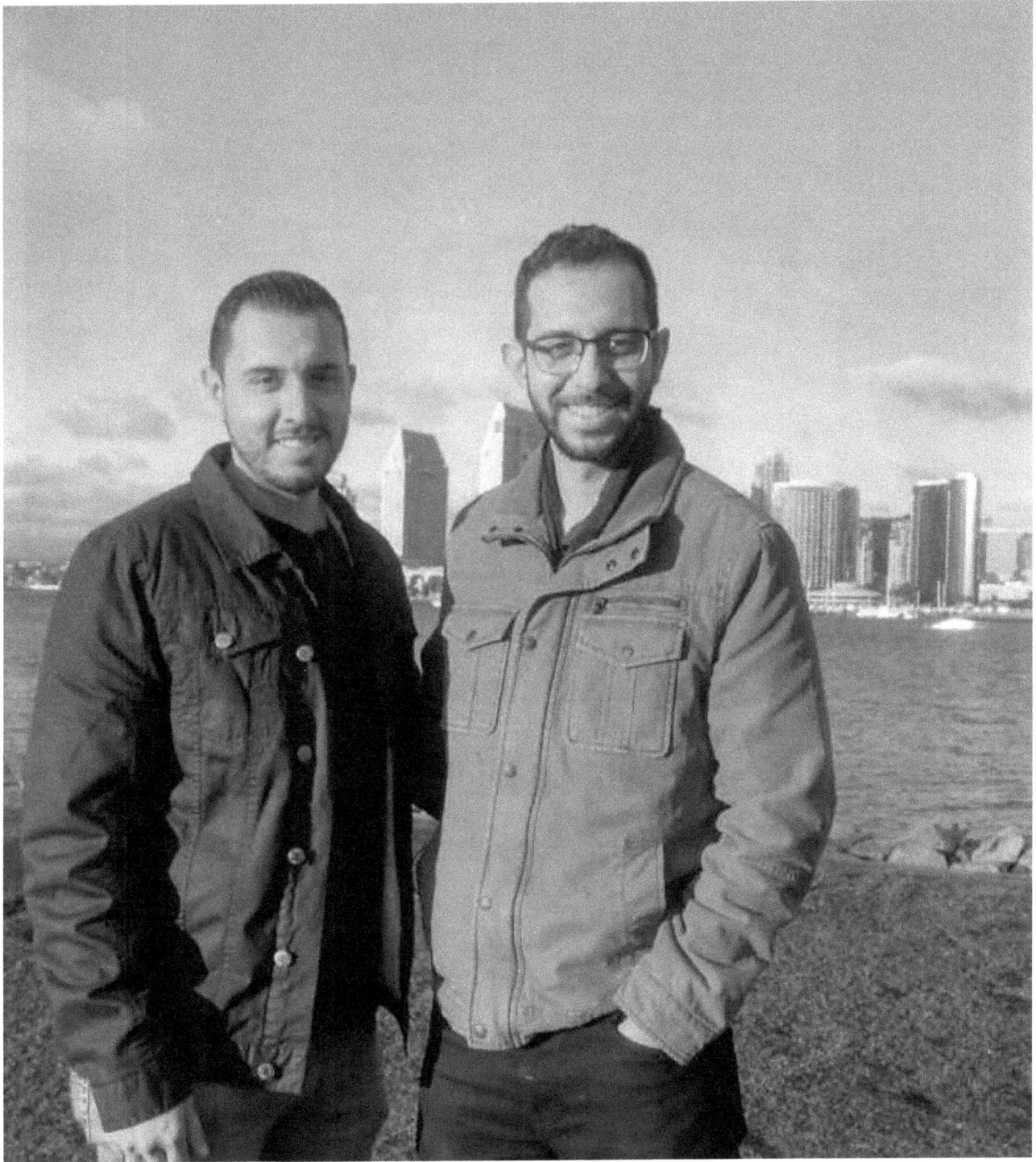

THE COOLEST BROTHERS

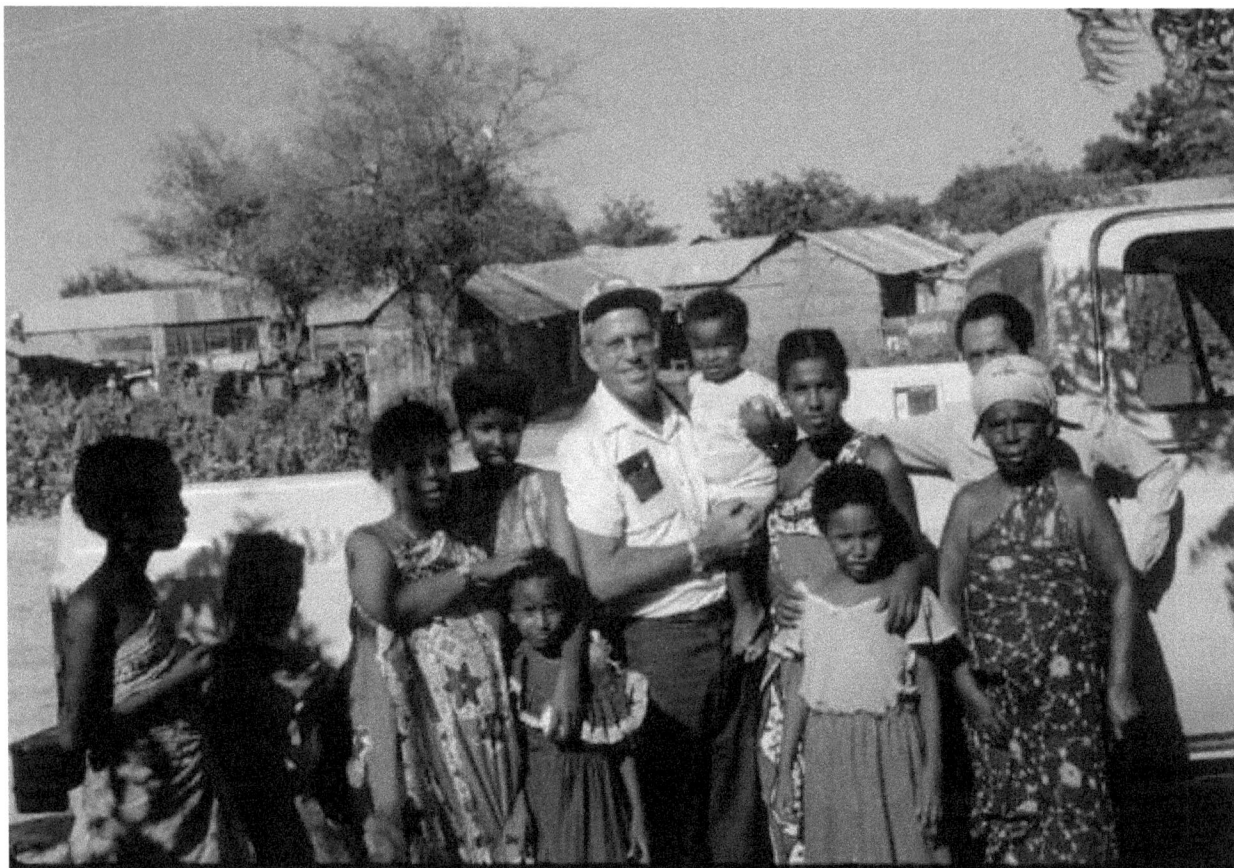

BEN LINDSAY WITH RURAL SOMALIS
KINDNESS KNOWS NO COLOR

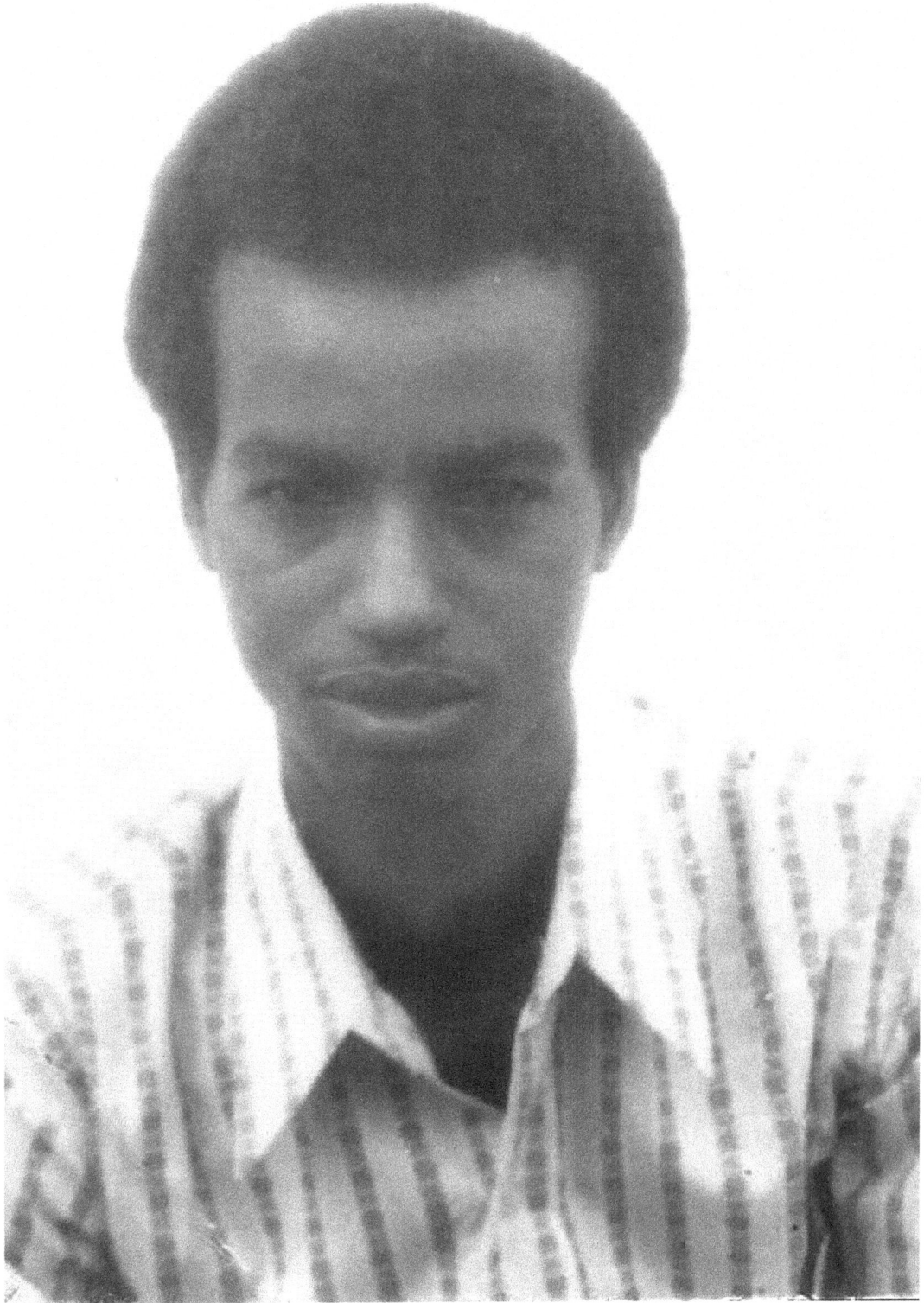

ALI ABDULAHI IBRAHIM
FROM JAMAMA TOWN
FRIENDS FOR LIFE

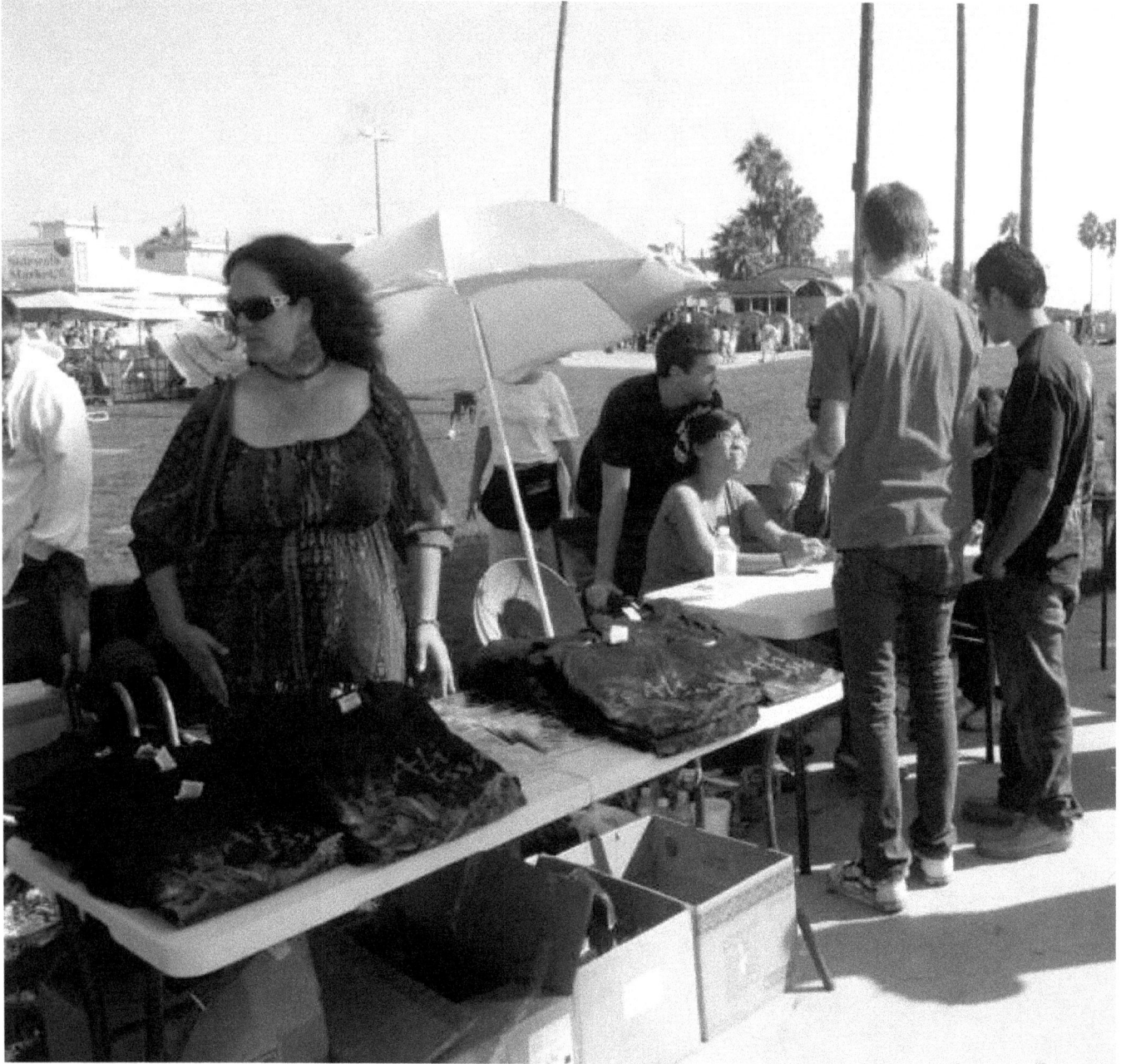

MY T-SHIRTS WERE
POPULAR AT VENICE BEACH, CALIFORNIA

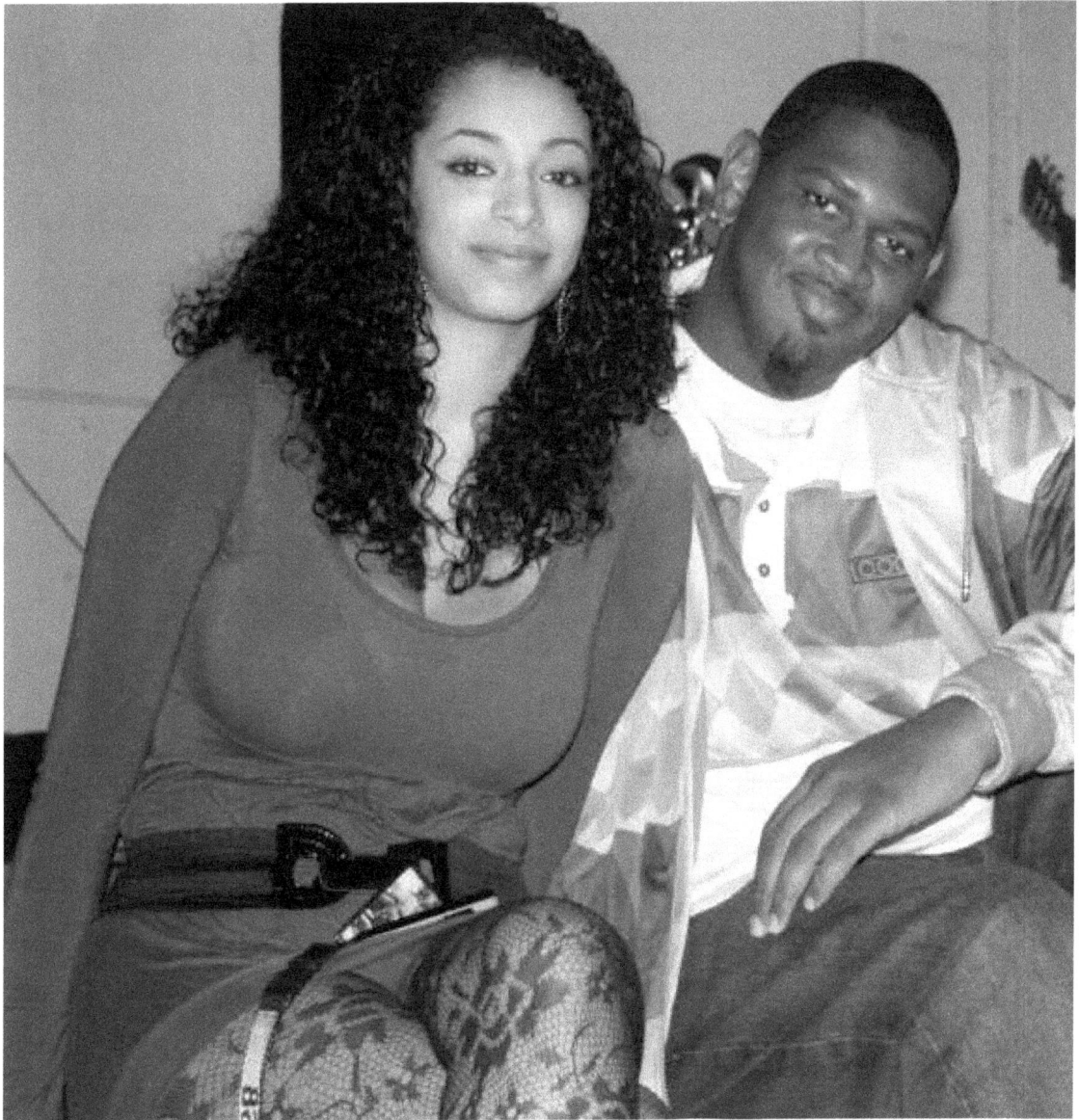

THEY ALWAYS LIGHTEN UP THE PARTY

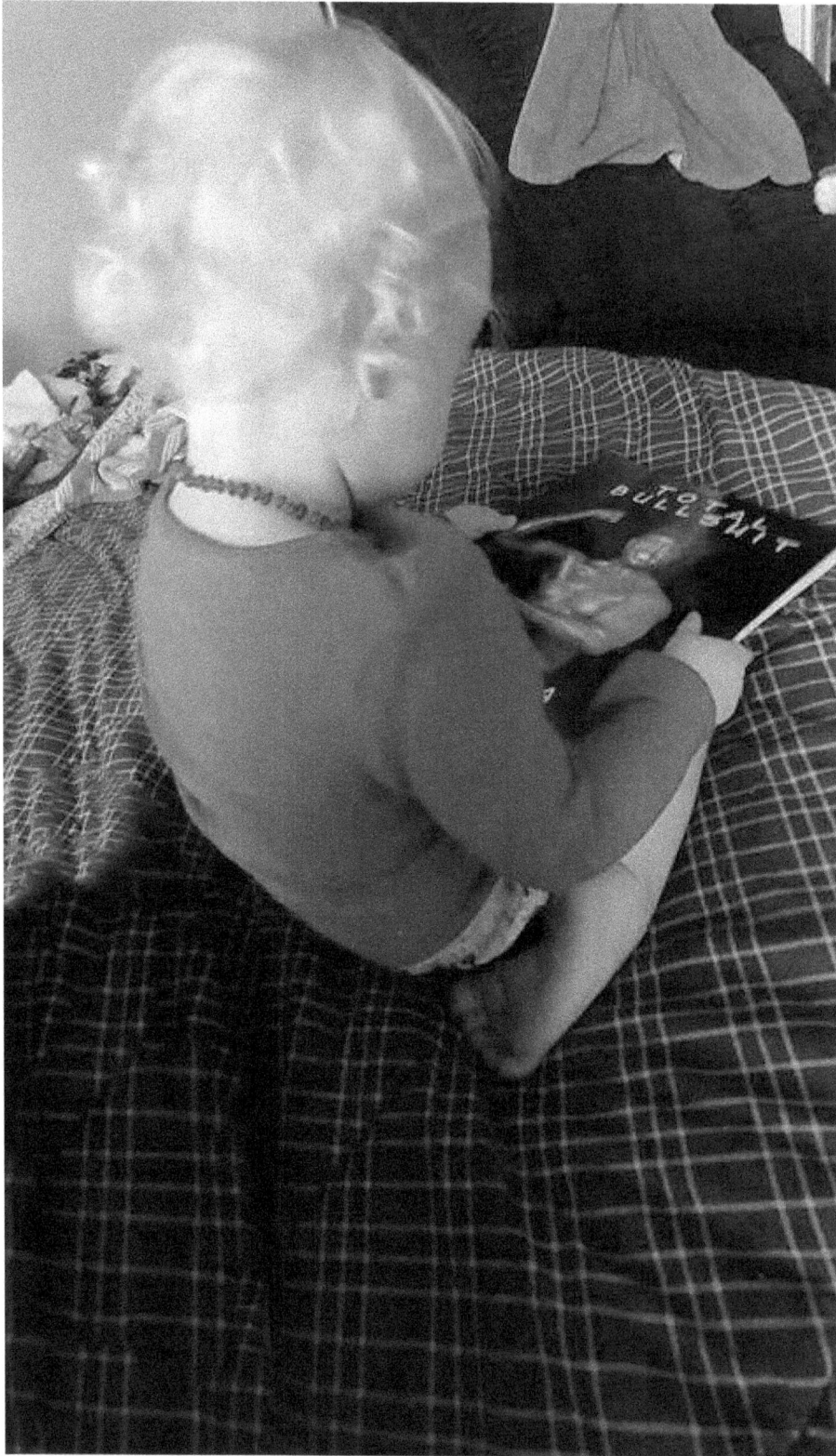

SHE WAS BORN TO READ AND BE A
FUTURISTIC WRITER

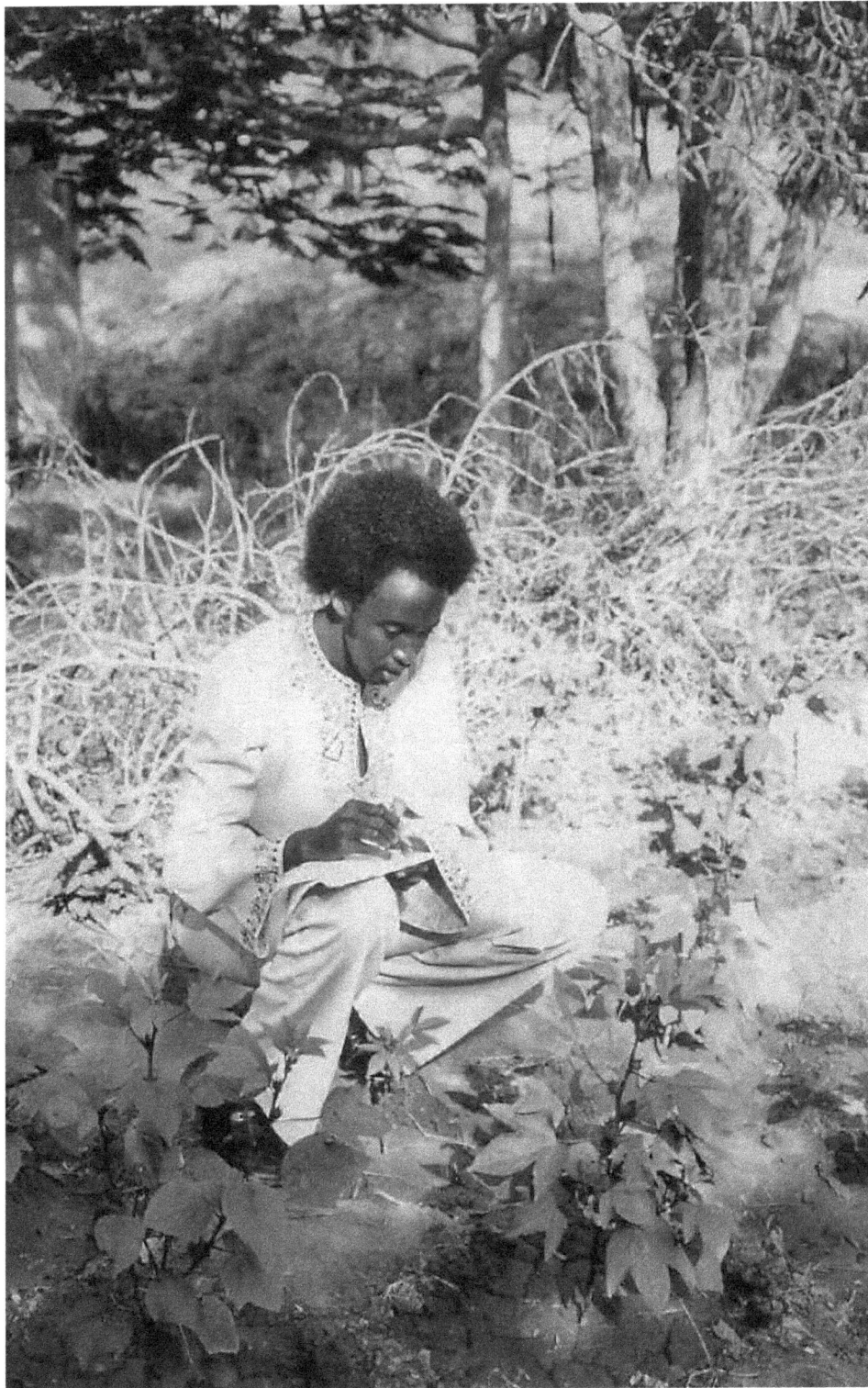

I INTRODUCED CANNABIS TO SOMALIA

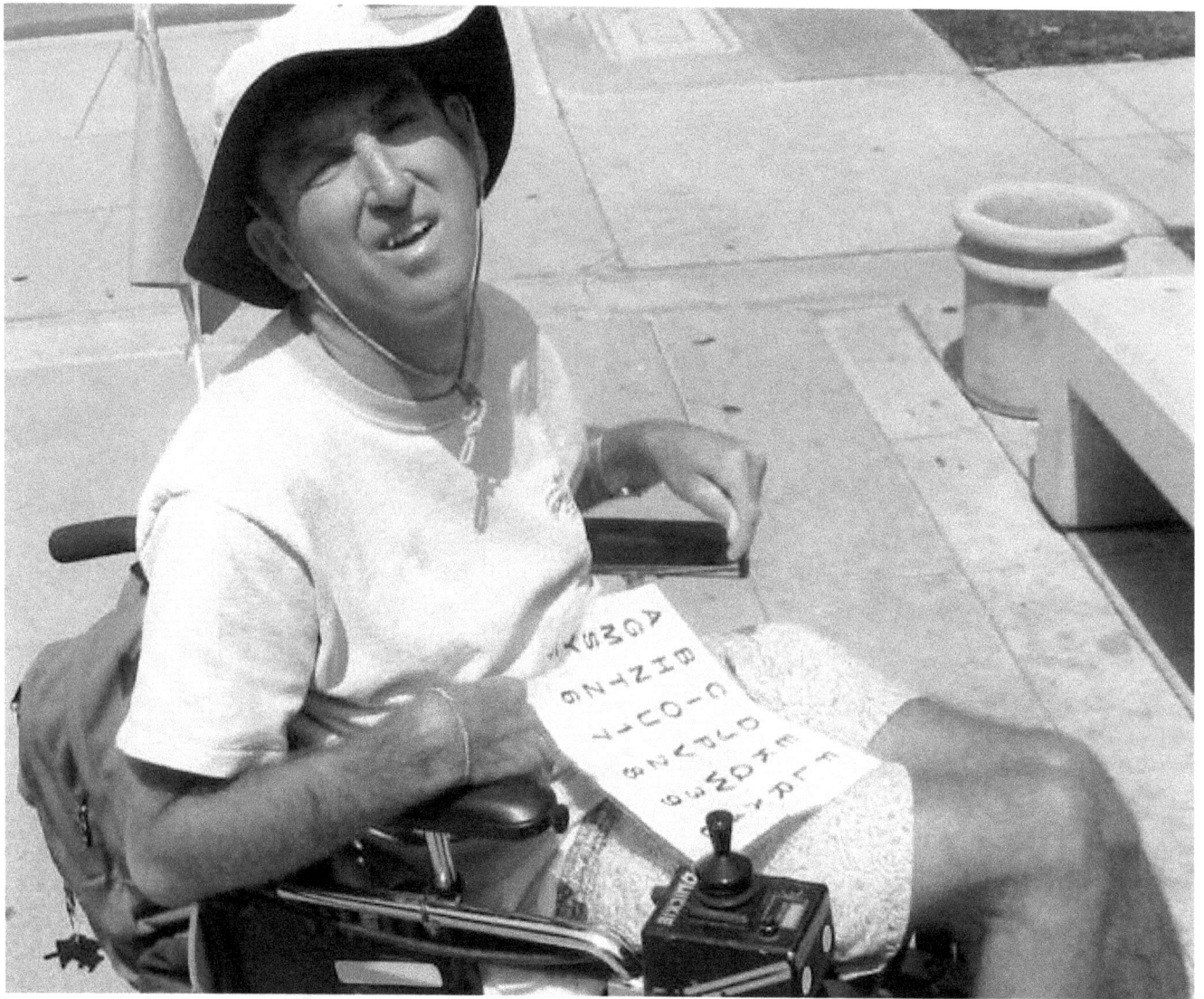

HE REFUSES TO GIVE UP, SO WHY
SHOULD ANYONE ELSE?

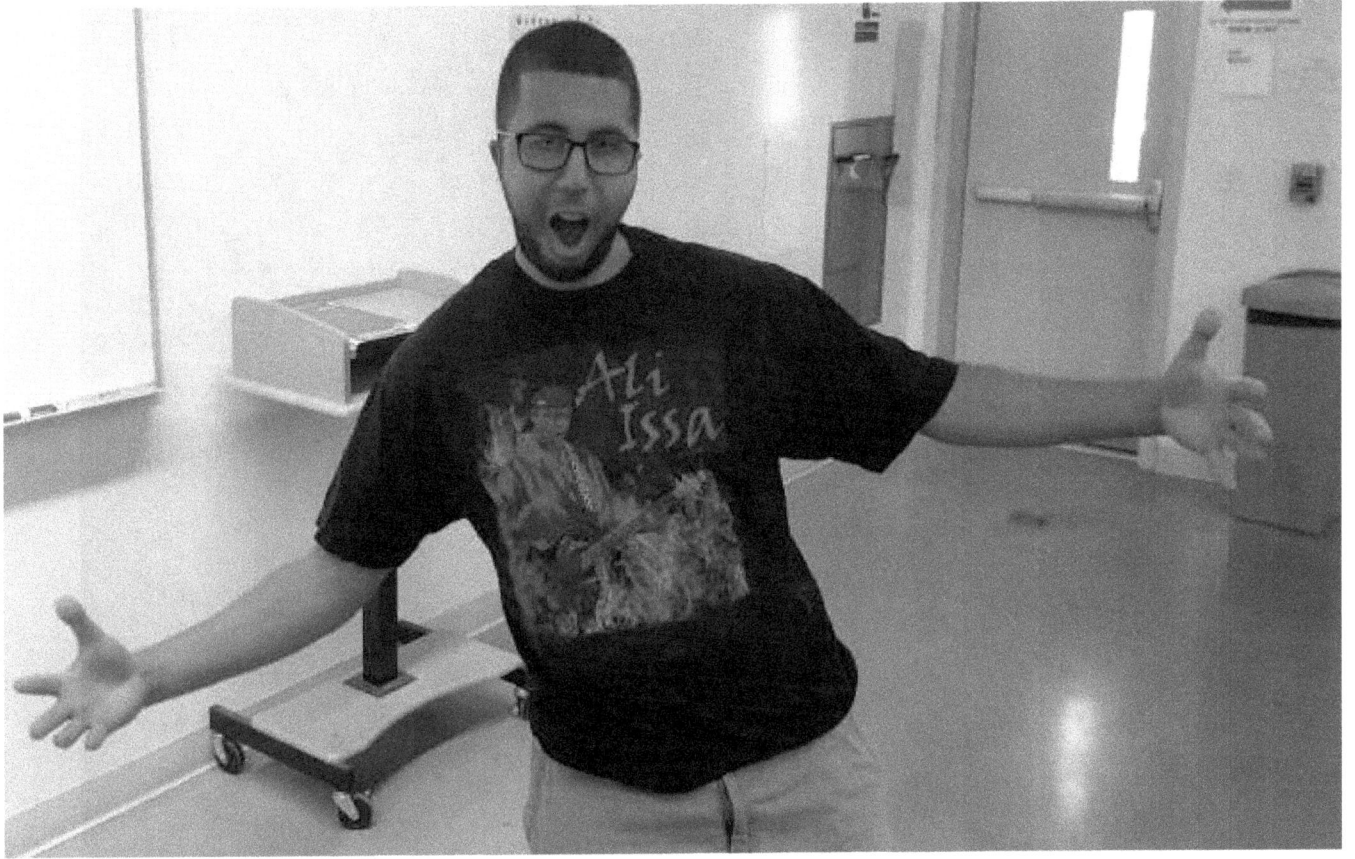

THEY CALL HIM DRIZZY
STAYS CURRENT ON THE RAP MUSIC

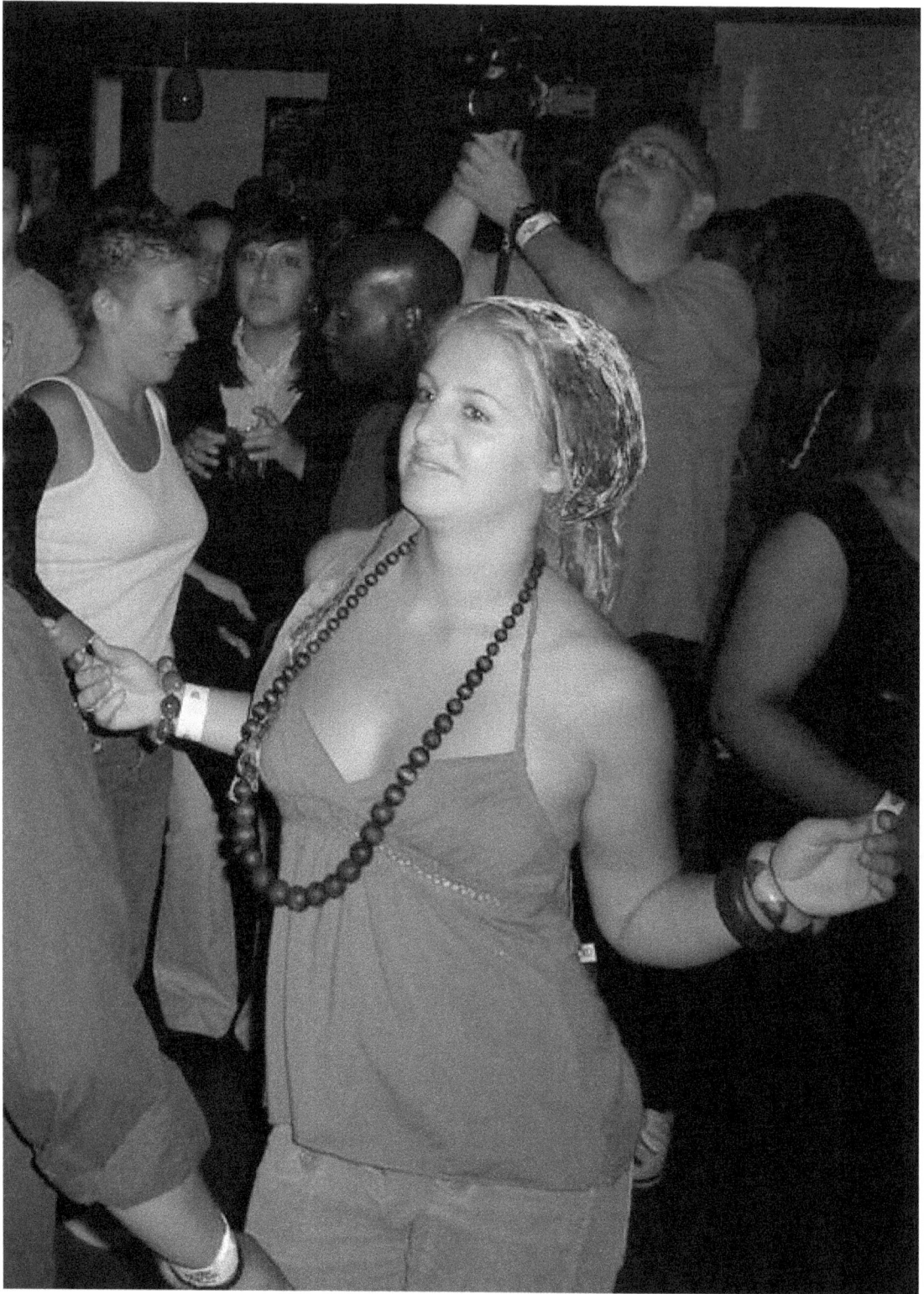

THE REGGAE LADY WAS COLORFUL AND
SPLIFFY

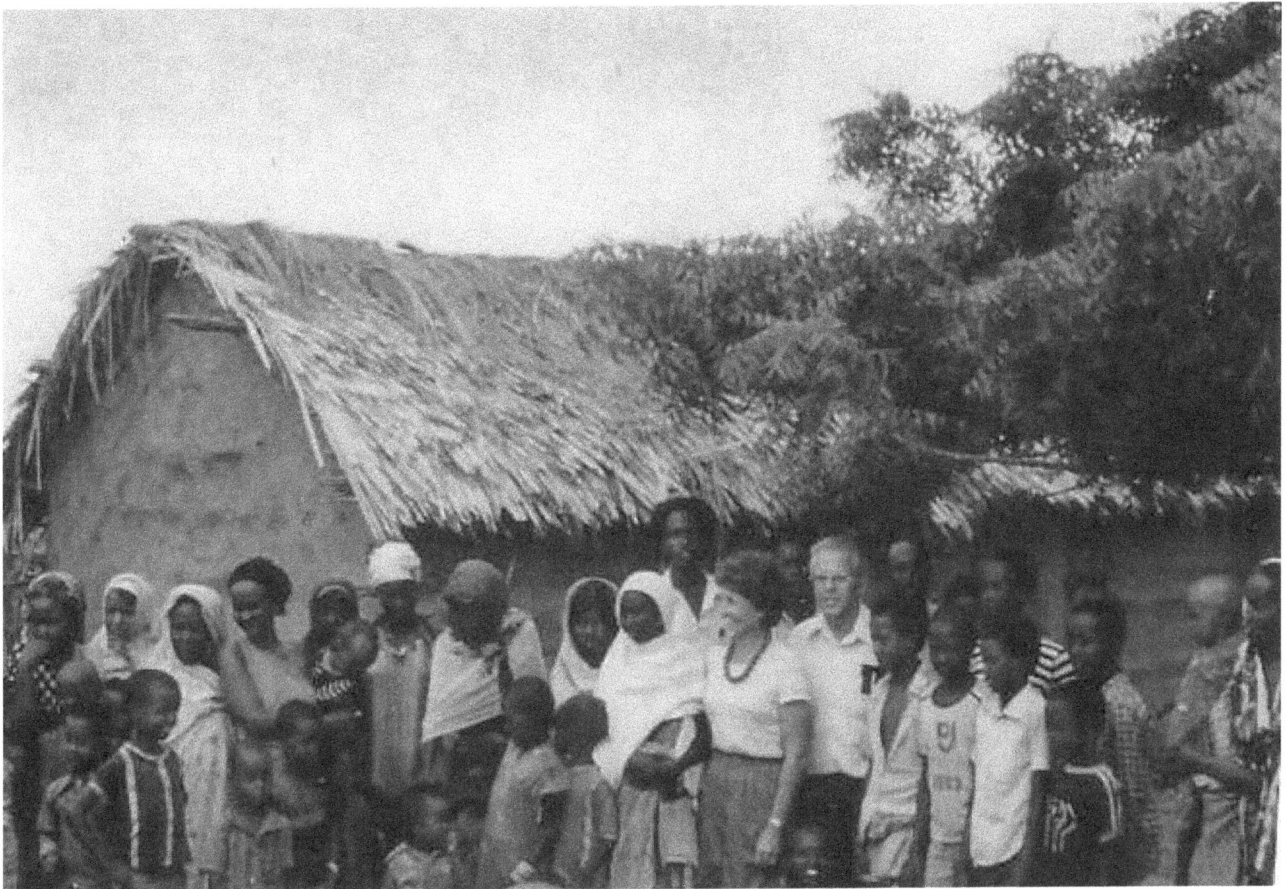

JAMAMA TOWN
MY HOUSE IS MADE OUT OF
PALM LEAVES, STICKS, AND
PLASTERED WITH MUD AND COW MANURE

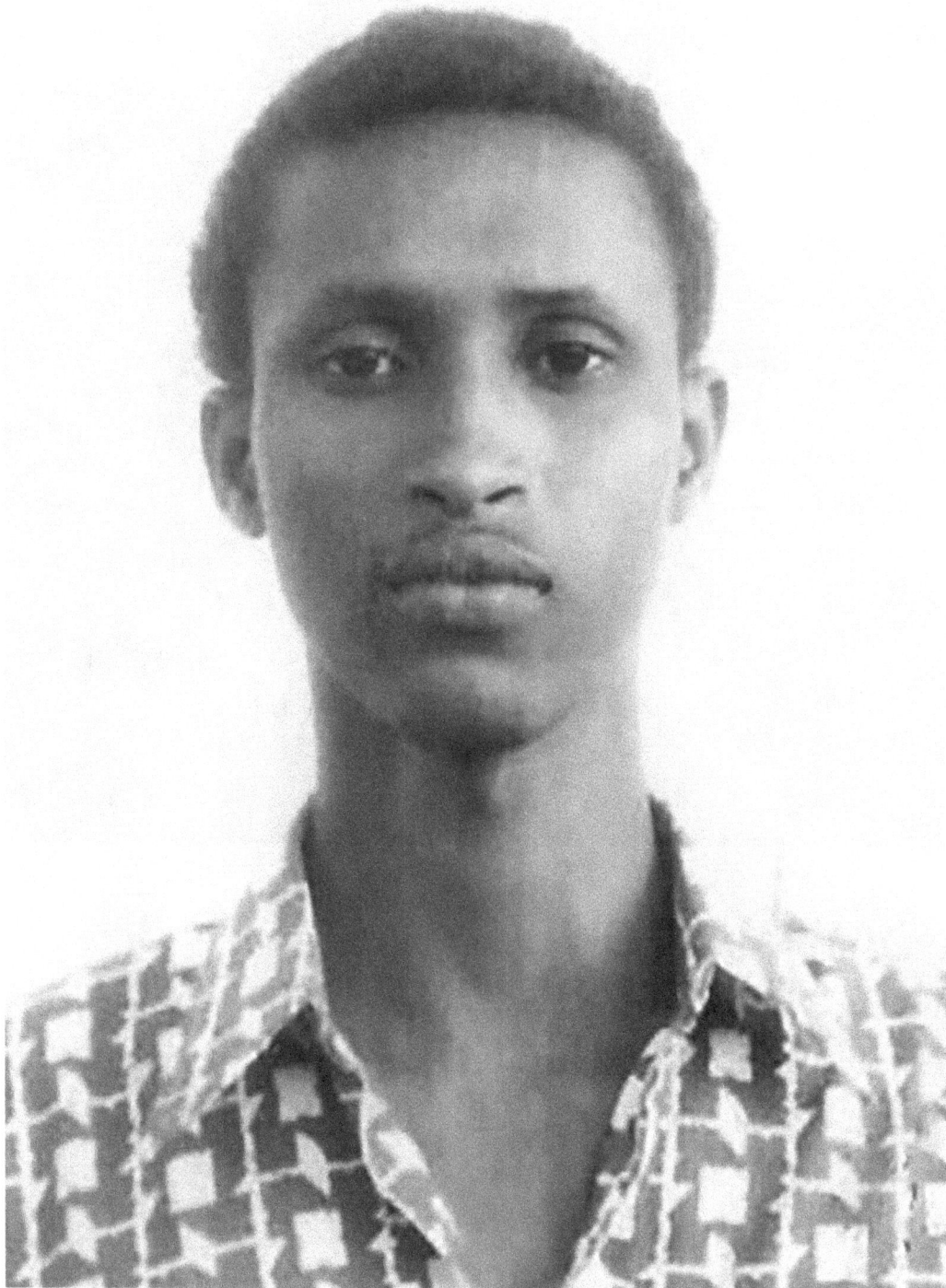

MOHAMED FARAH FROM JELIB TOWN
EDUCATED IN JAMAMA TOWN

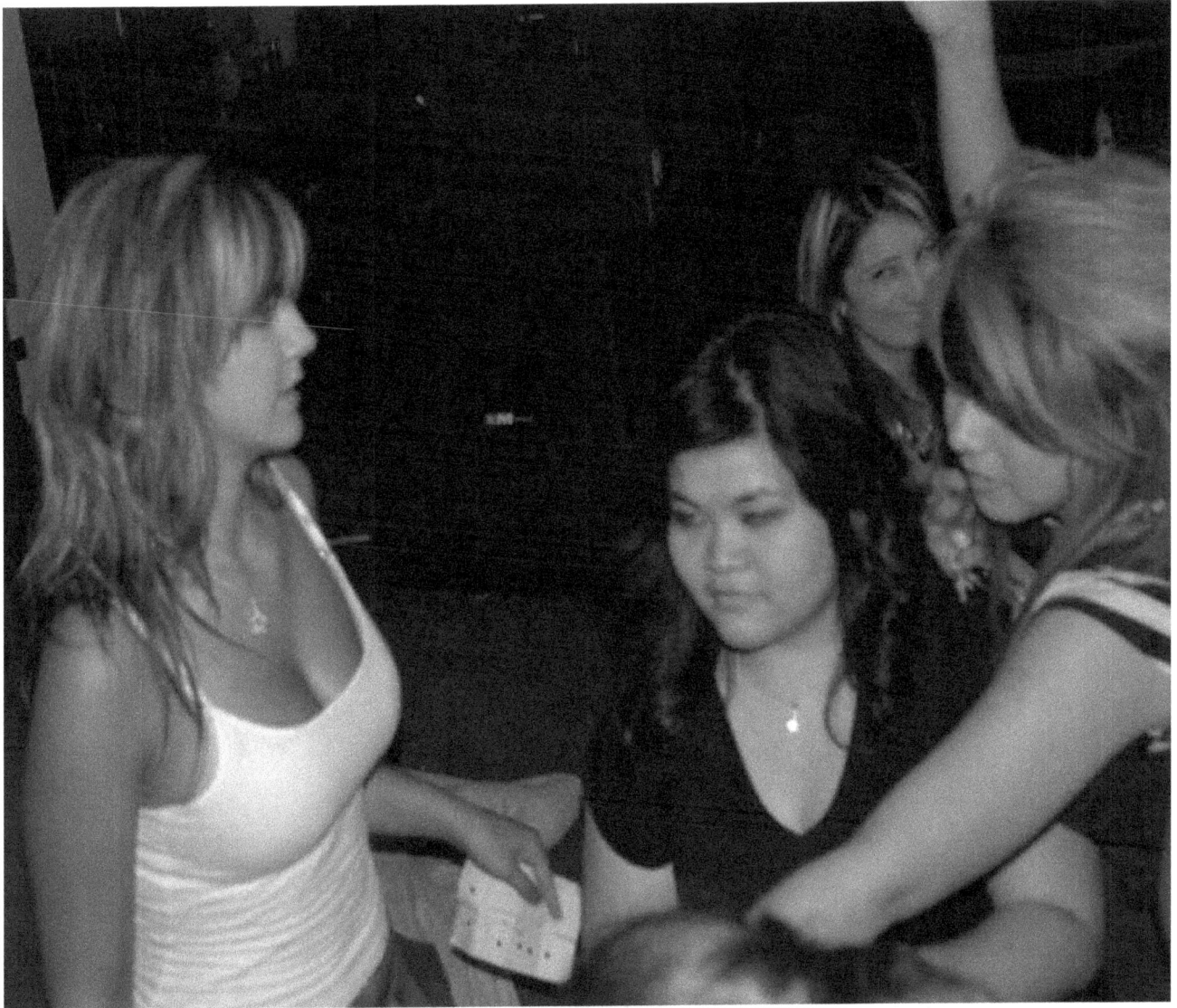

WOMEN CHECK OUT EACH OTHER
ALL THE TIME

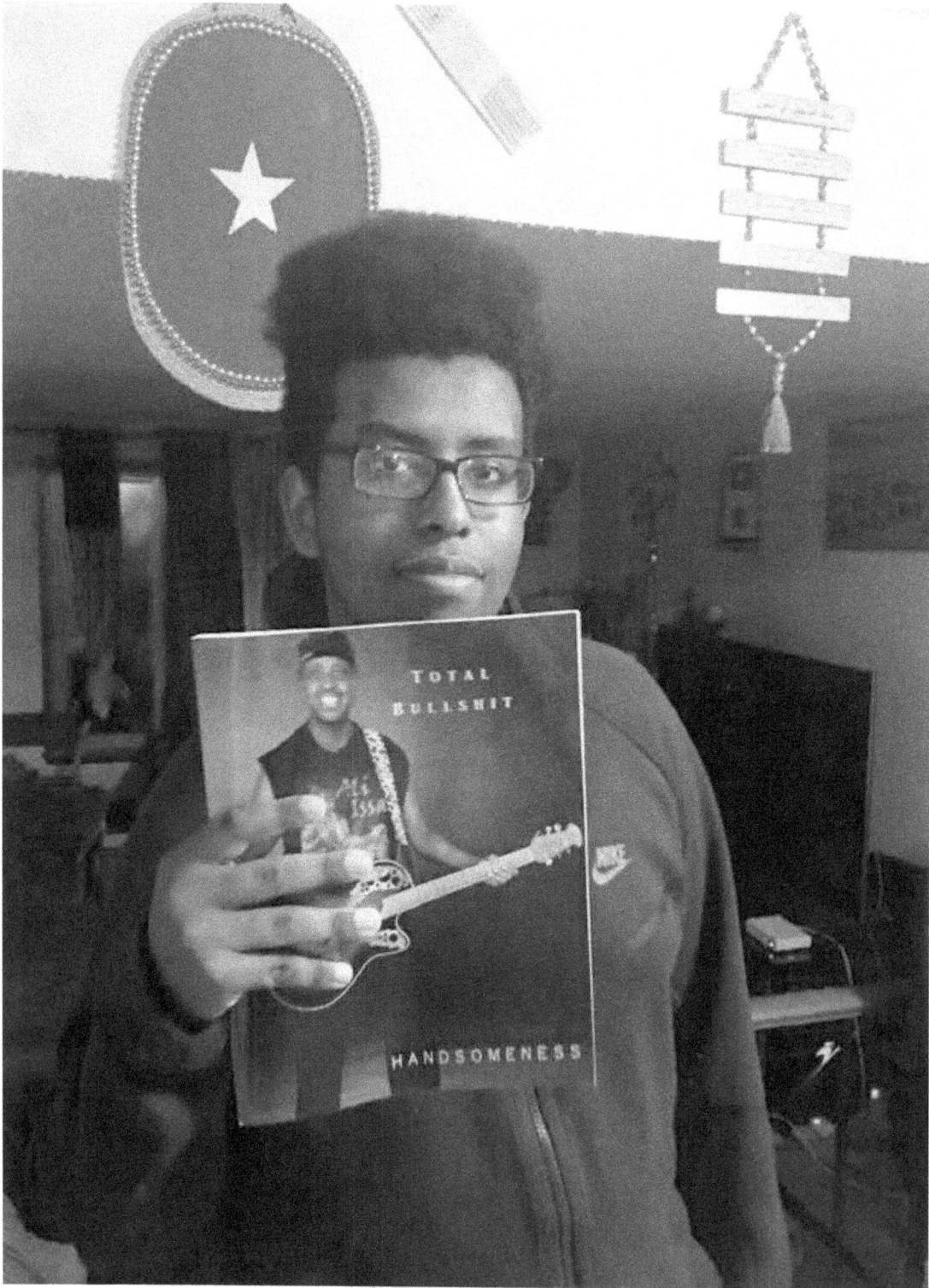

THE ROBLE FAMILY
MADE MY FIRST BOOK POPULAR

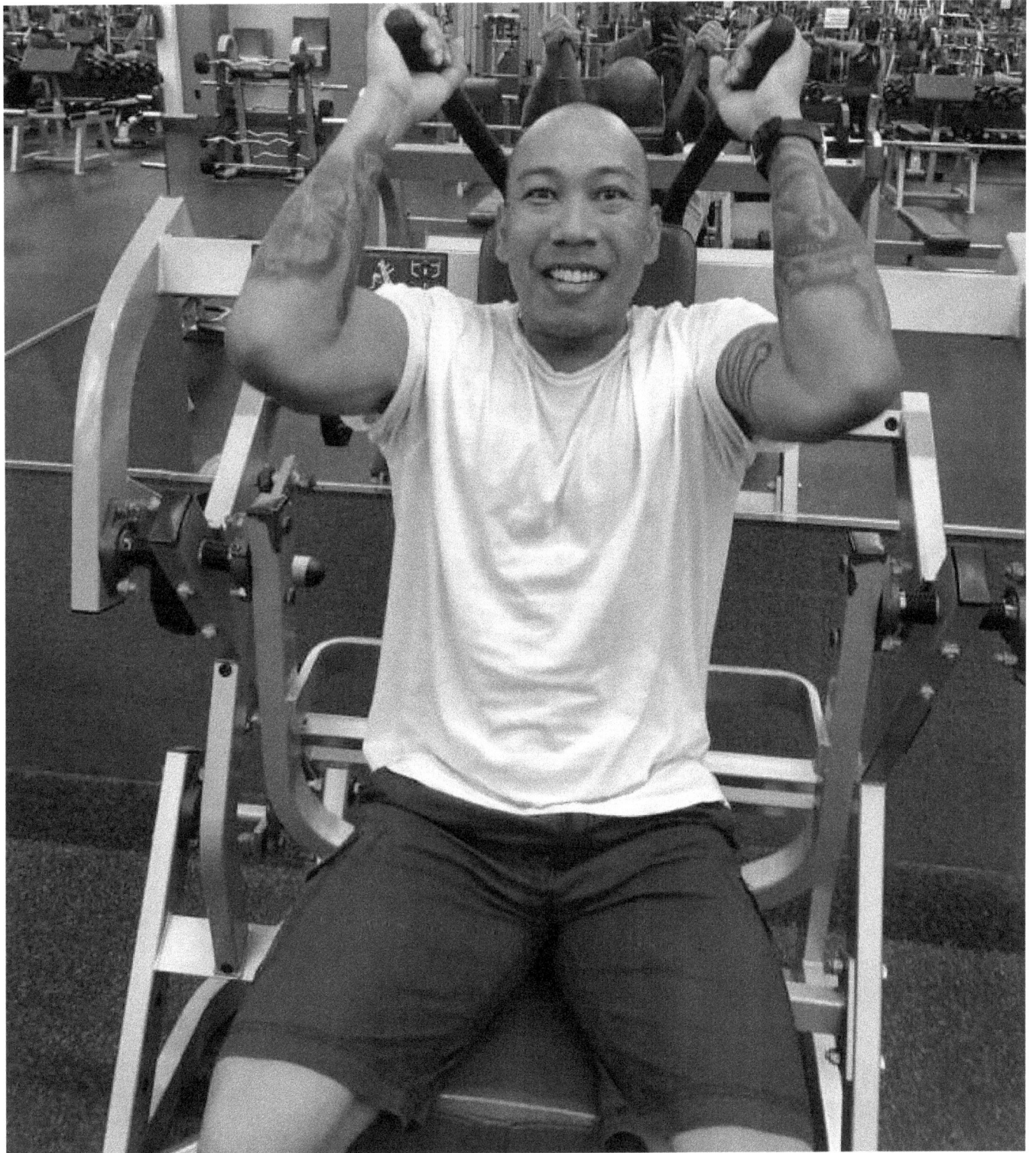

THE BLAZING HASHISH MAN

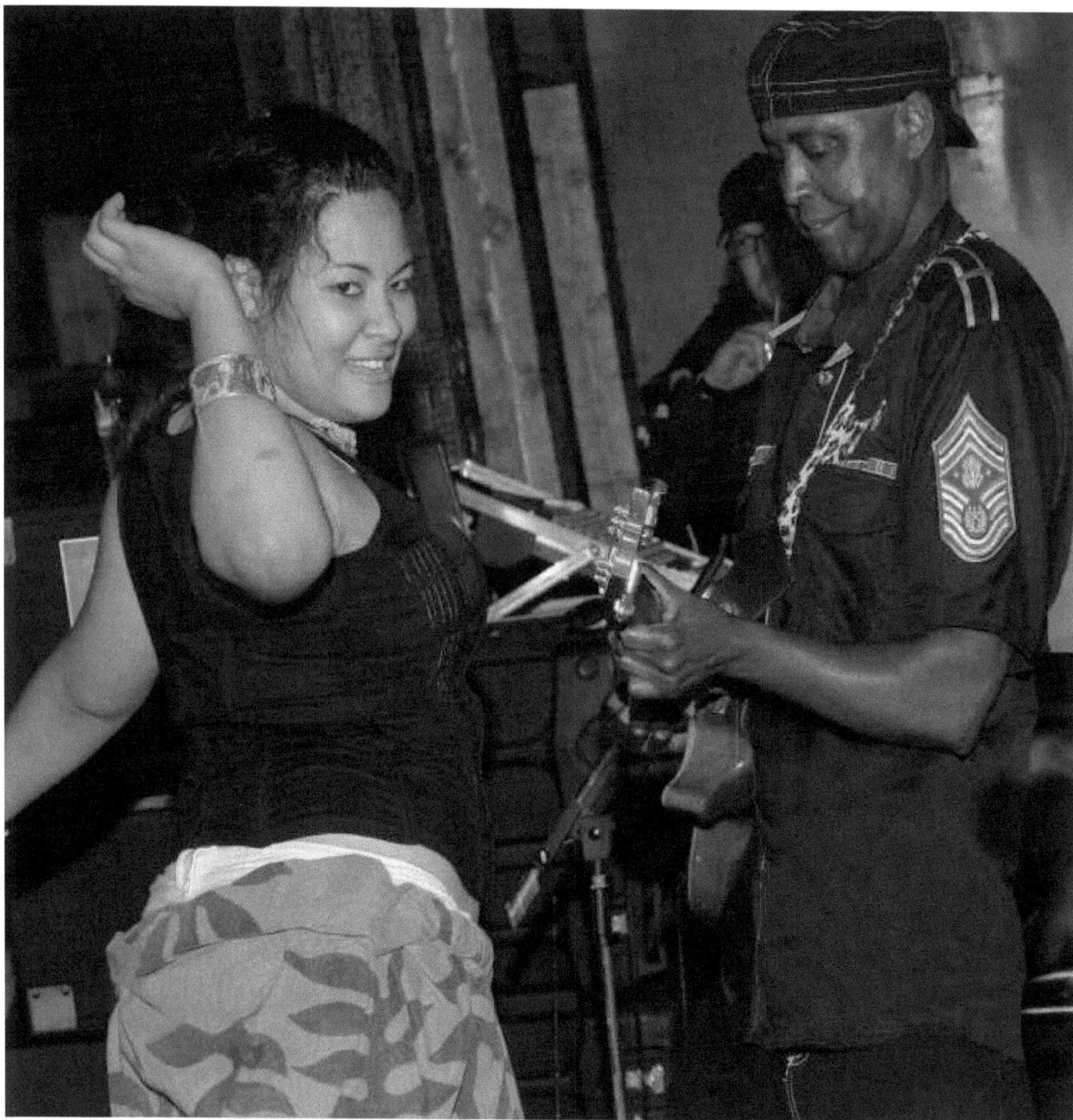

THE GUITAR SOUNDS MAKES HER MOVE

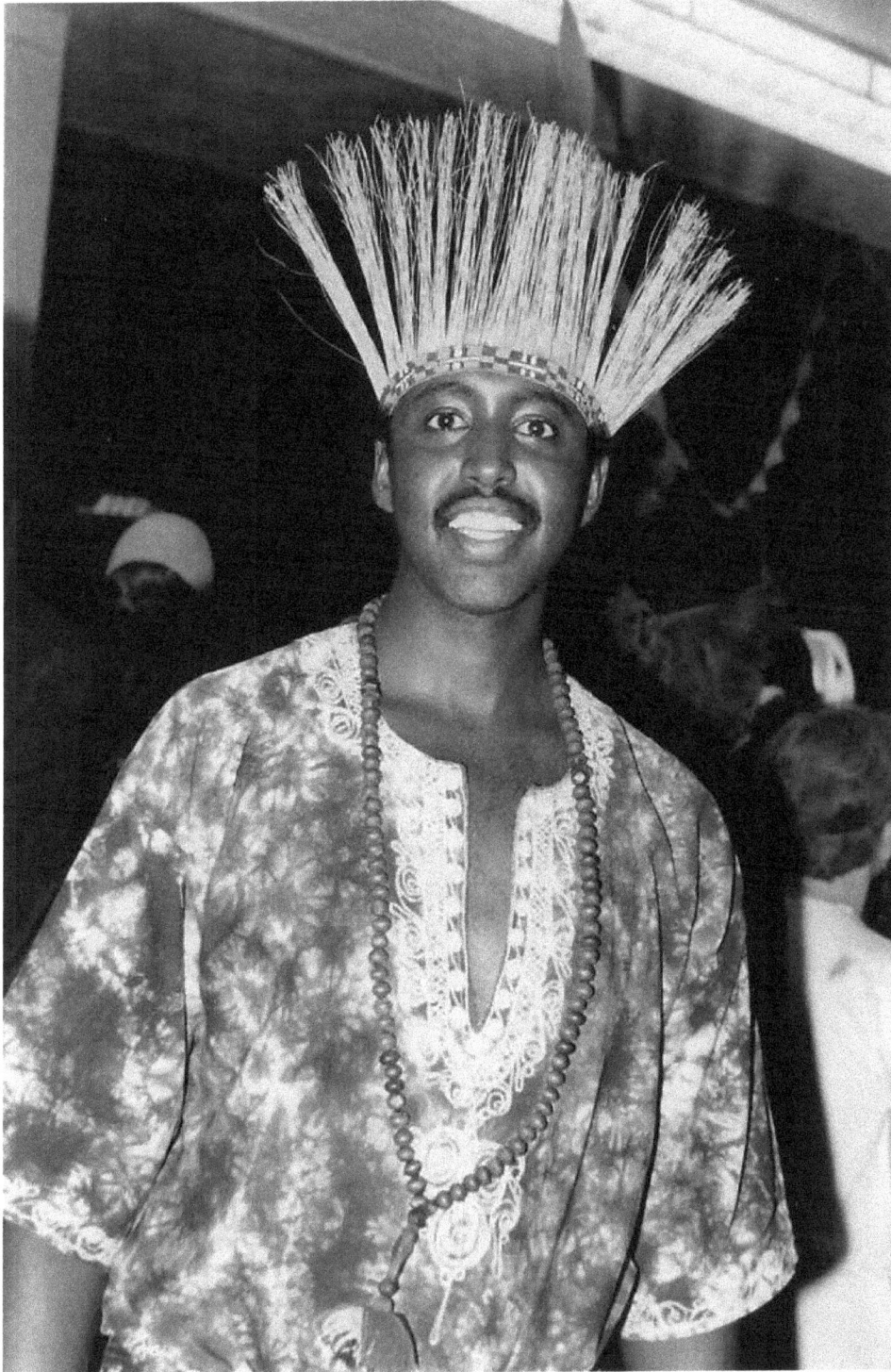

REPRESENTING THE TRADITION
OF MY HOME COUNTRY

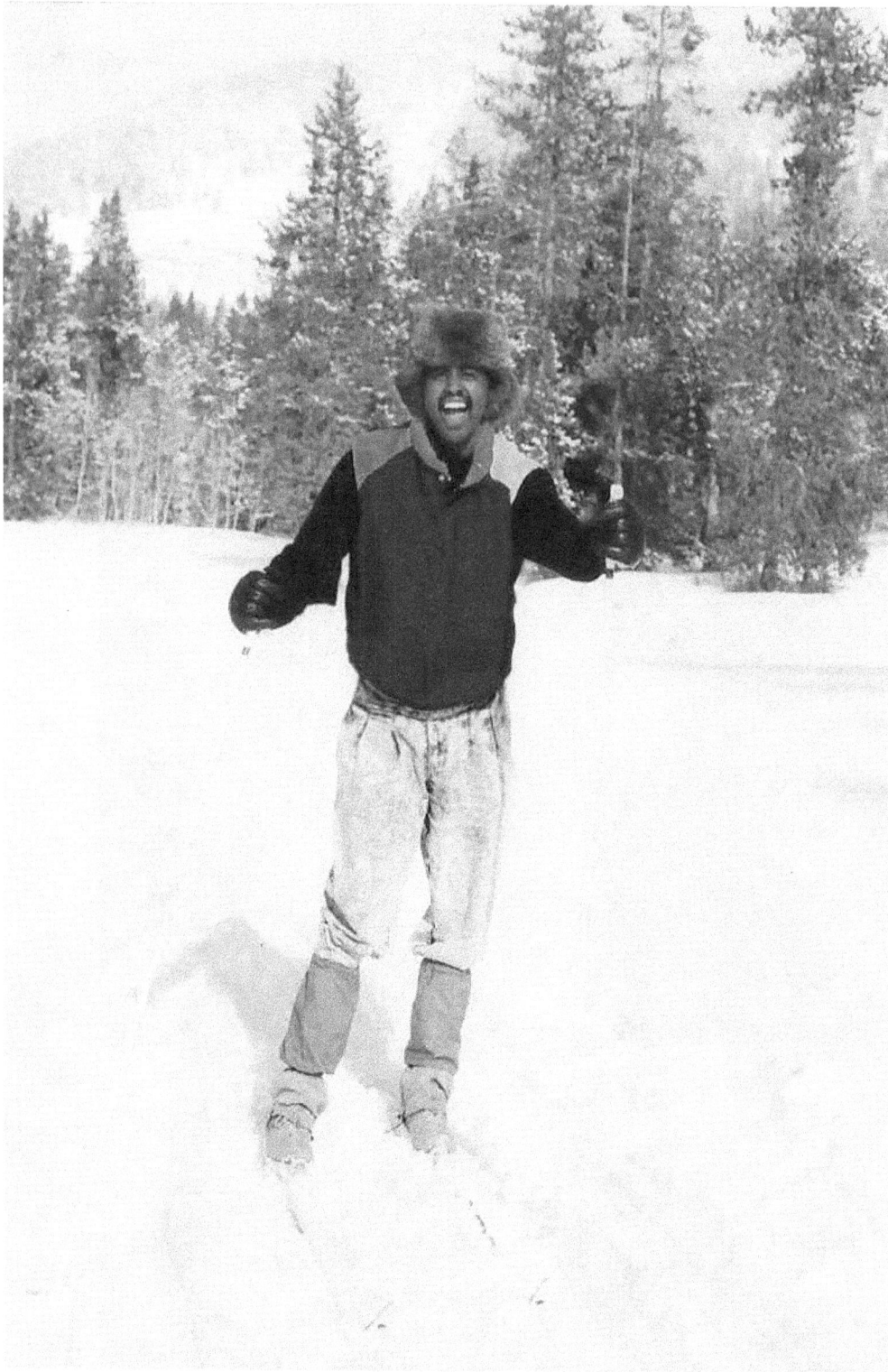

EVERY TIME I FALL,
I AM BACK ON MY FEET

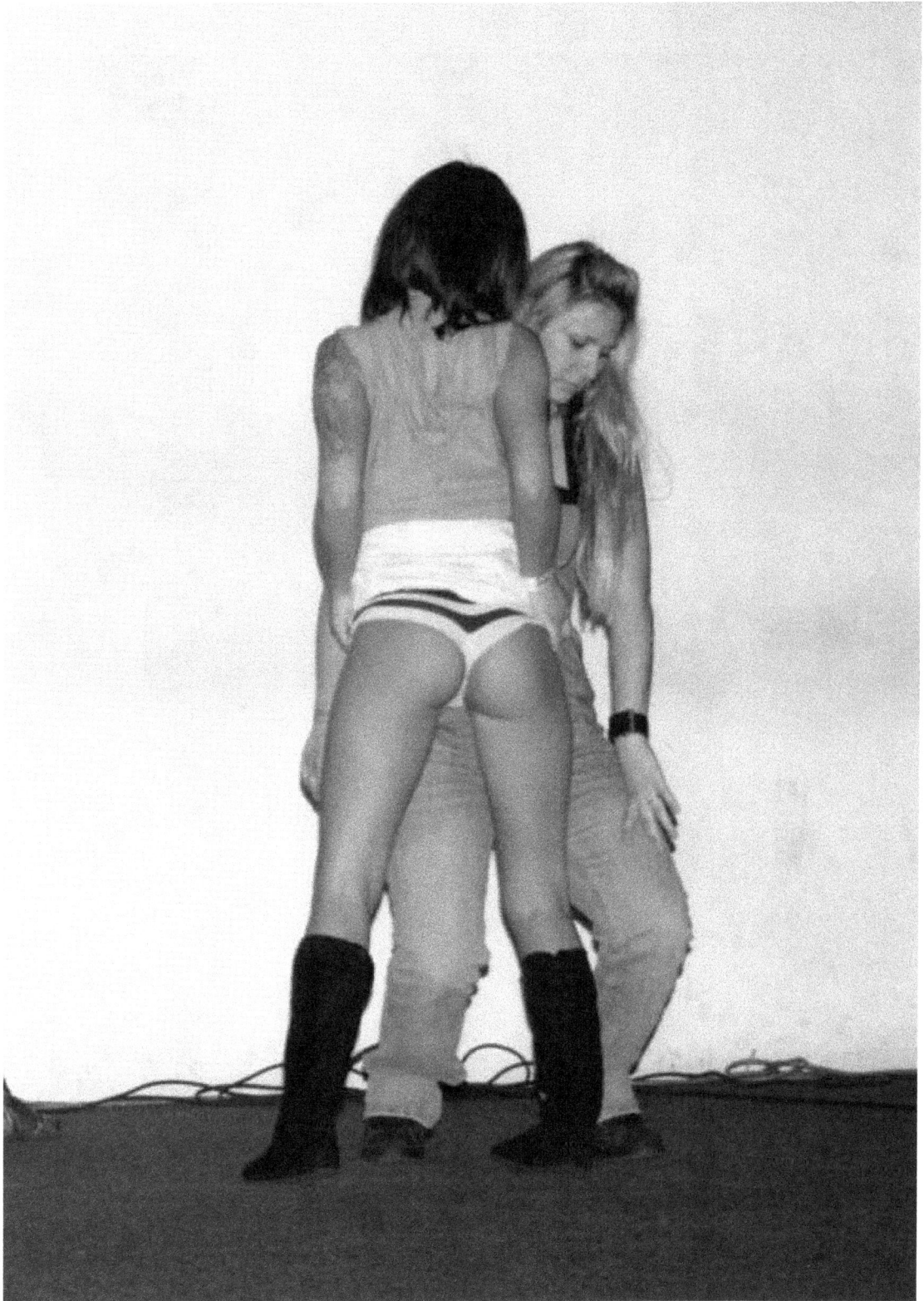

THE NASTIER THEY DANCED
THE BETTER I PLAYED THE MUSIC

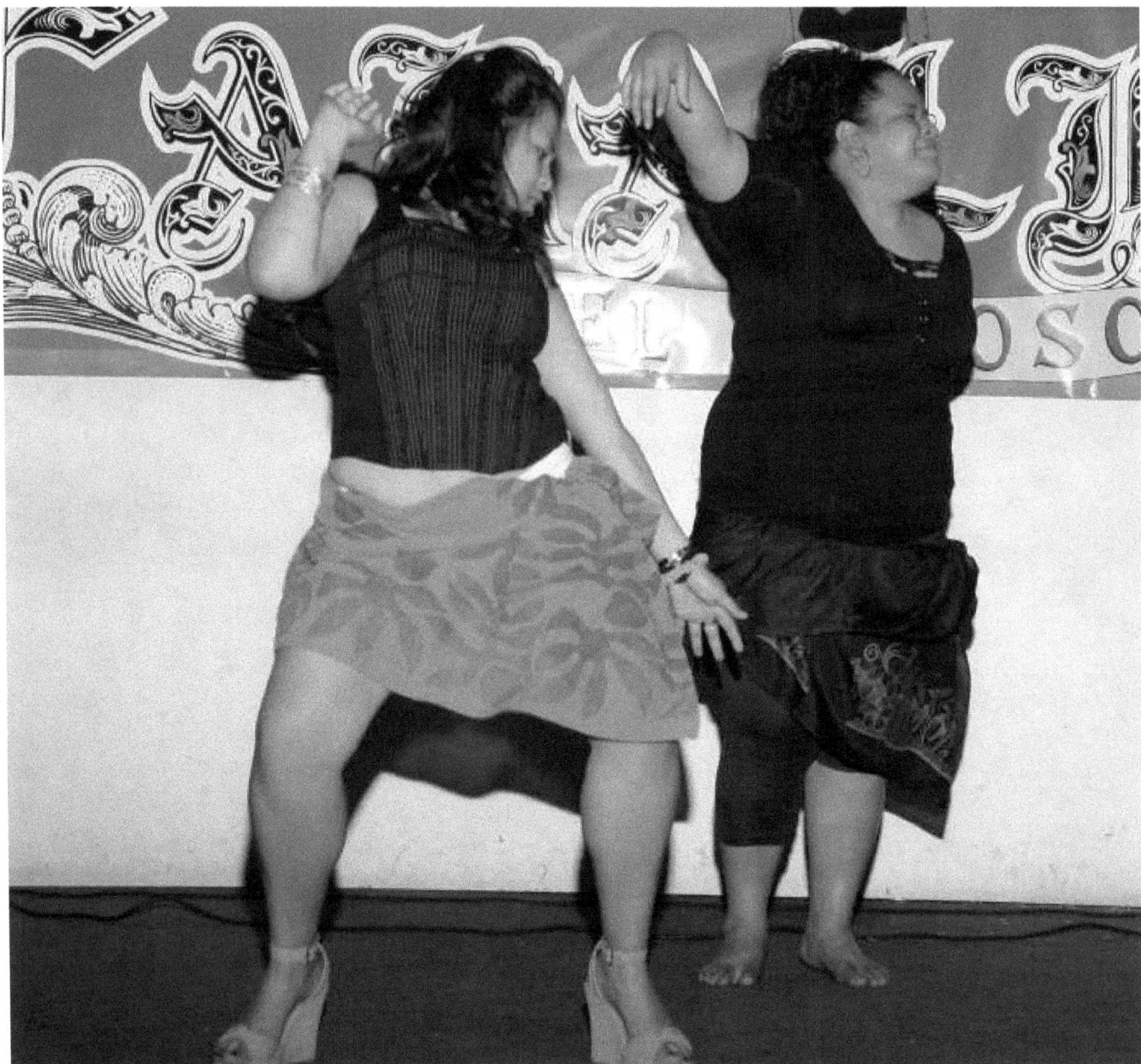

THE ISLAND GIRLS SET
MY SOUL ON FIRE

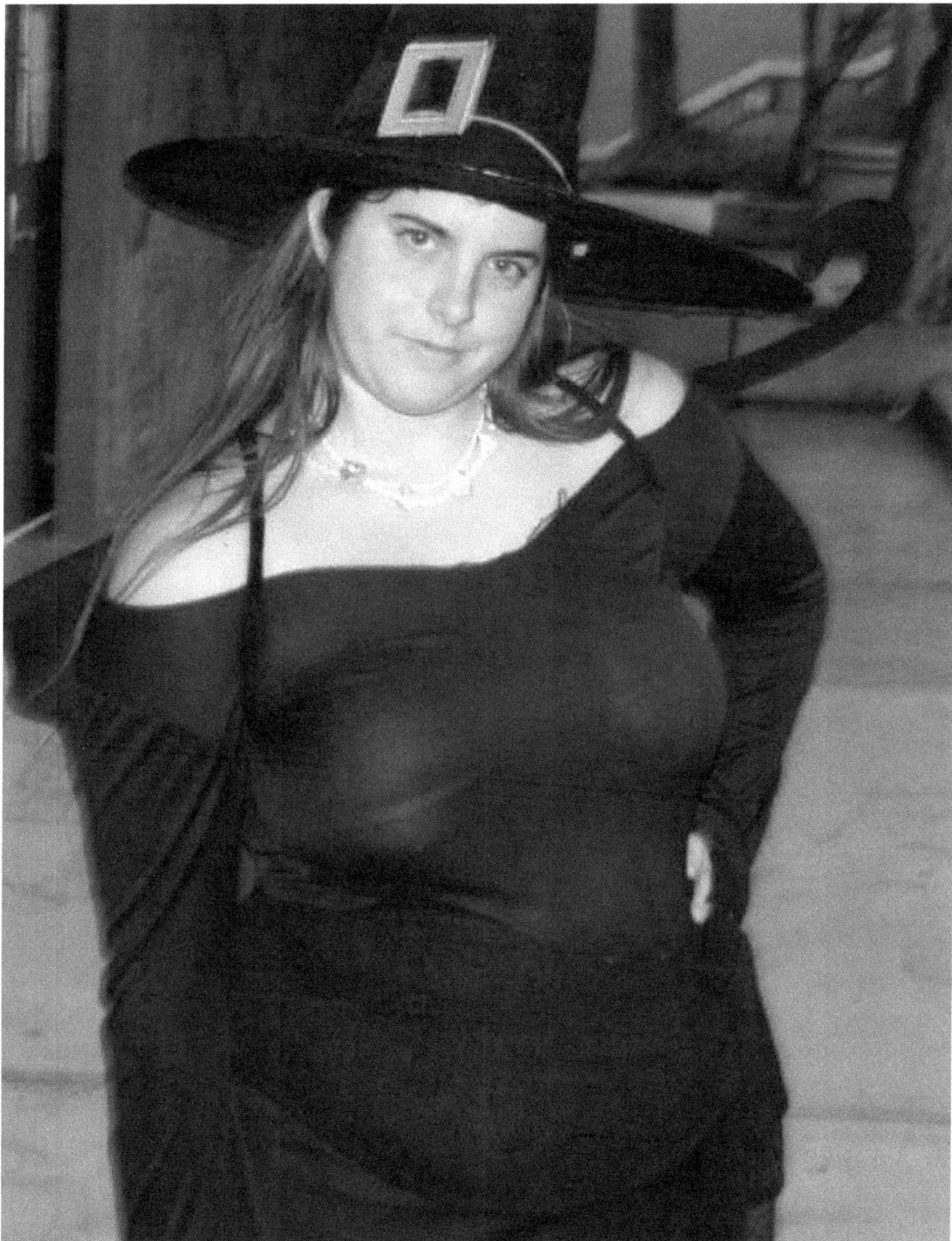

I AM VERY DISTRACTED

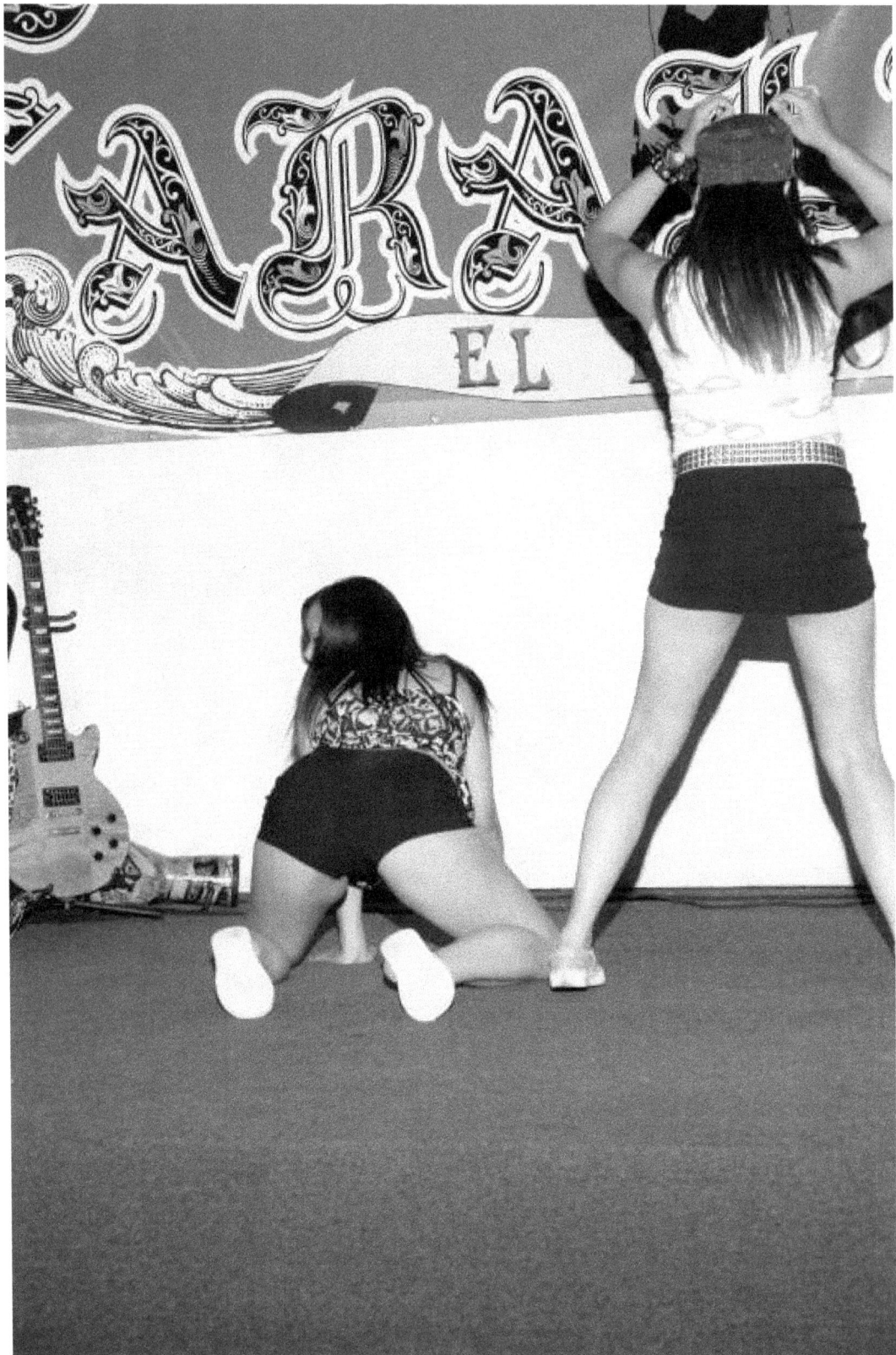

THEIR MOVES GOT
THE CROWD GO CRAZY

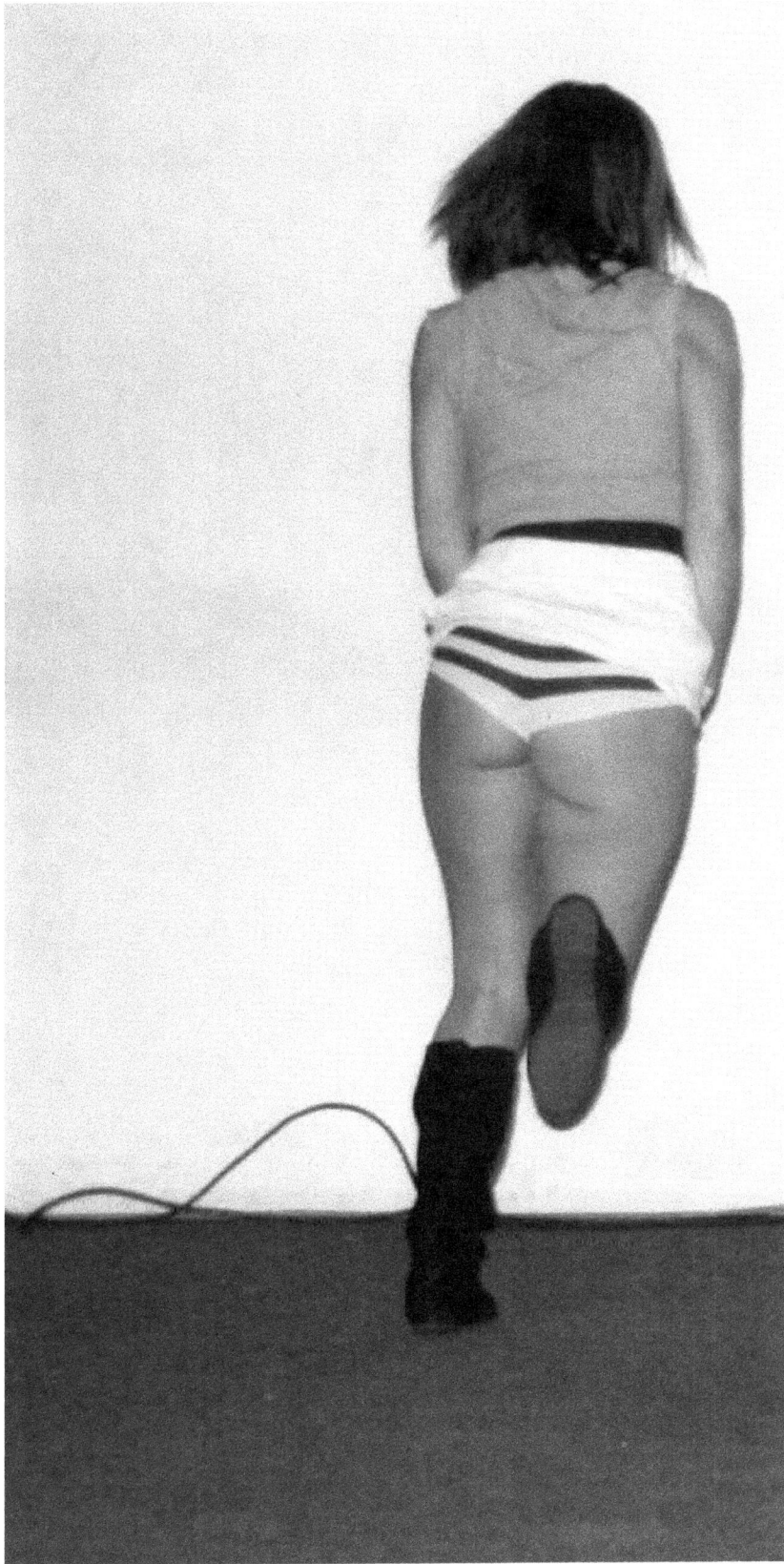

FREE SPIRIT DANCING LADY

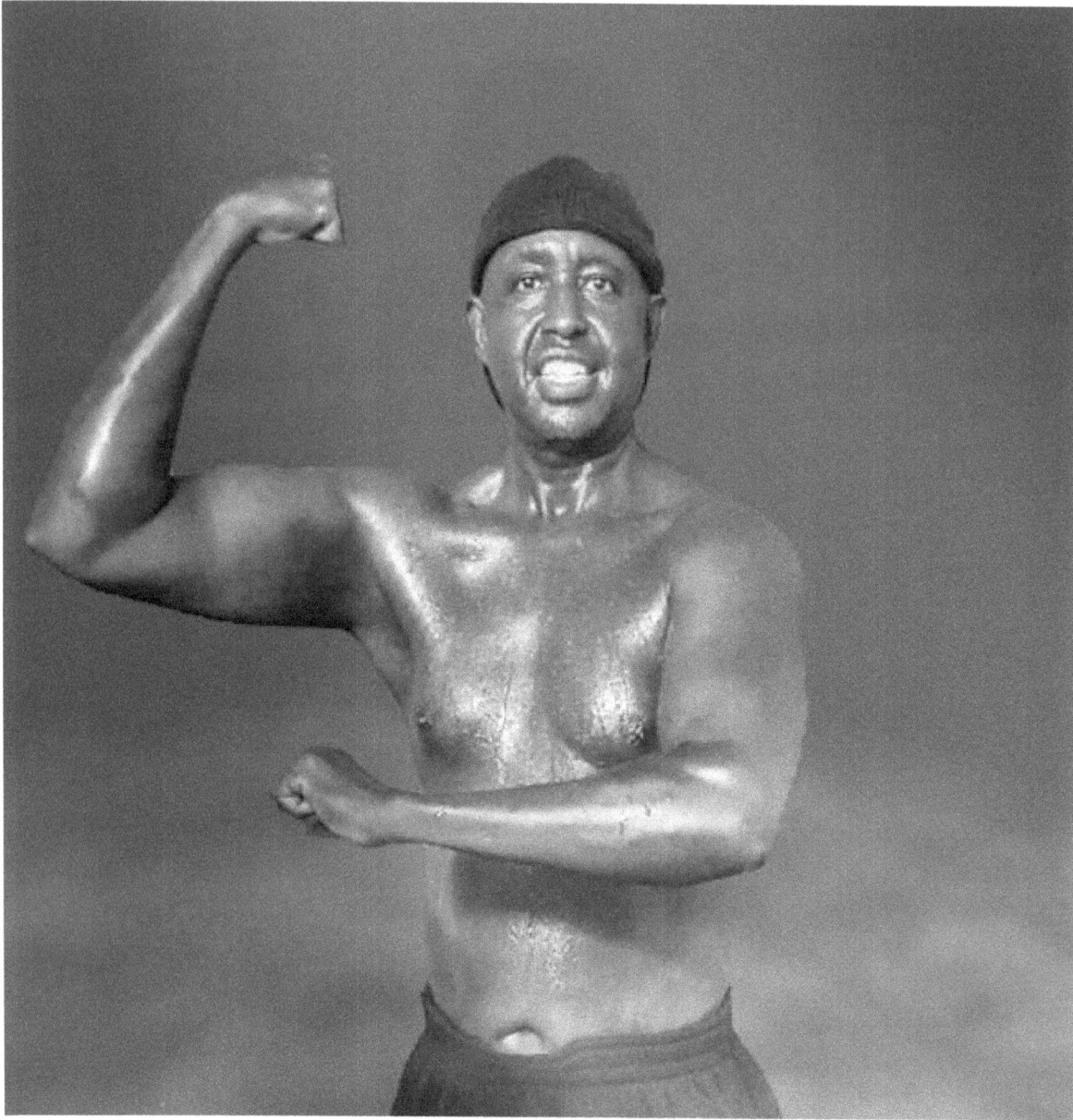

WHEN YOUR MIND IS STRONG,
YOUR BODY, SOUL, AND SPIRIT
WILL BE STRONGER

THANKS TO ALL THE PEOPLE WHO
MAKE MY BOOKS POPULAR.
I APPRECIATE YOUR
UNCONDITIONAL SUPPORT.